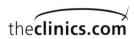

theclinics.com

PSYCHIATRIC CLINICS
OF NORTH AMERICA

Bipolar Disorder

GUEST EDITOR
E. Sherwood Brown, MD, PhD

June 2005 • Volume 28 • Number 2

SAUNDERS

An Imprint of Elsevier, Inc.
PHILADELPHIA   LONDON   TORONTO   MONTREAL   SYDNEY   TOKYO

W.B. SAUNDERS COMPANY
A Division of Elsevier Inc.

The Curtis Center • Independence Square West • Philadelphia, Pennsylvania 19106

http://www.theclinics.com

THE PSYCHIATRIC CLINICS OF NORTH AMERICA	Volume 28, Number 2
June 2005	ISSN 0193-953X
Editor: Sarah E. Barth	ISBN 1-4160-2679-7

The Psychiatric Clinics of North America (ISSN 0193-953X) is published quarterly by the W.B. Saunders Company. Corporate and editorial offices: 1600 JFK Boulevard, Suite 1800, Philadelphia, PA 19103-2822. Accounting and circulation offices: 6277 Sea Harbor Drive, Orlando, FL 32887-4800. Periodicals postage paid at Orlando, FL 32862, and additional mailing offices. Subscription prices are $170.00 per year (US individuals), $288.00 per year (US institutions), $85.00 per year (US students/residents), $205.00 per year (Canadian individuals), $349.00 per year (Canadian Institutions), $240.00 per year (foreign individuals), $349.00 per year (foreign institutions), and $120.00 per year (international & Canadian students/residents). Foreign air speed delivery is included in all *Clinics'* subscription prices. All prices are subject to change without notice. POSTMASTER: Send address changes to *The Psychiatric Clinics of North America*, W.B. Saunders Company, Periodicals Fulfillment, Orlando, FL 32887—4800. **Customer Service: 1-800-654-2452 (US). From outside of the US, call 1-407-345-4000.**

The Psychiatric Clinics of North America is covered in *Index Medicus, Current Contents/Social and Behavioral Sciences, Social Science Citation Index, Embase/Excerpta Medica,* and PsycINFO.

Printed in the United States of America.

GUEST EDITOR

E. SHERWOOD BROWN, MD, PhD, Assistant Professor and Director, Psychoneuroendocrine Research Program, Department of Psychiatry, University of Texas Southwestern Medical Center, Dallas, Texas

CONTRIBUTORS

MATTEO BALESTRIERI, MD, Professor of Psychiatry, Section of Psychiatry, Department of Pathology and Experimental & Clinical Medicine, University of Udine; and InterUniversity Center for Behavioral Neurosciences, University of Udine, Udine, Italy

PAOLO BRAMBILLA, MD, Assistant Professor of Psychiatry, Section of Psychiatry, Department of Pathology and Experimental & Clinical Medicine, University of Udine; and Coordinator, Verona-Udine Brain Imaging Program, InterUniversity Center for Behavioral Neurosciences, University of Udine, Udine, Italy

E. SHERWOOD BROWN, MD, PhD, Assistant Professor and Director, Psychoneuroendocrine Research Program, Department of Psychiatry, University of Texas Southwestern Medical Center, Dallas, Texas

JOSEPH R. CALABRESE, MD, Professor of Psychiatry and Co-Director, Bipolar Disorder Research Center, Case University School of Medicine; Director, Mood Disorders Program; and Director, Division of Ambulatory Care, University Hospitals of Cleveland, Cleveland, Ohio

FRANCESC COLOM, D CLIN PSYCH, PhD, Clinical Psychologist, Department of Psychiatry, Bipolar Disorders Research Program, Stanley Centre for Bipolar Disorders Research, Barcelona, Spain; and Visiting Senior Lecturer, Institute of Psychiatry, De Crespigny Park, Denmark Hill, London, UK

C. MUNRO CULLUM, PhD, Professor of Psychiatry and Neurology, Departments of Psychiatry and Neurology, The University of Texas Southwestern Medical Center at Dallas, Dallas, Texas

C. DABAN, PhD, Neuropsychologist and Research Fellow, Bipolar Disorders Program, Hospital Clinic, University of Barcelona, Barcelona, Spain

MELISSA P. DELBELLO, MD, Associate Professor of Psychiatry and Pediatrics, University of Cincinnati Medical Center, Cincinnati, Ohio; Department of Psychiatry, Cincinnati Children's Hospital Medical Center, Cincinnati, Ohio

J. RAYMOND DEPAULO, JR, MD, Henry Phipps Professor and Director, Department of Psychiatry and Behavioral Sciences, Johns Hopkins School of Medicine, Baltimore, Maryland

STEVEN L. DUBOVSKY, MD, Professor and Chairman, Department of Psychiatry, State University of New York at Buffalo, Buffalo, New York; and Adjunct Professor of Psychiatry and Medicine, University of Colorado, Denver, Colorado

AMELIA J. EISCH, PhD, Assistant Professor, Department of Psychiatry, University of Texas Southwestern Medical Center, Dallas, Texas

DAVID C. GLAHN, PhD, Assistant Professor of Psychiatry, Division of Schizophrenia and Related Disorders, Department of Psychiatry, University of Texas Health Science Center, San Antonio, Texas

ROBERT A. KOWATCH, MD, Professor of Psychiatry and Pediatrics, Cincinnati Children's Hospital Medical Center, Cincinnati, Ohio; Department of Psychiatry, University of Cincinnati Medical Center, Cincinnati, Ohio

DIANE C. LAGACE, PhD, Postdoctoral Research Fellow, Department of Psychiatry, University of Texas Southwestern Medical Center, Dallas, Texas

P. MACKIN, MB, BS, PhD, MRCPsych, Academic Specialist Registrar in Psychiatry, University of Newcastle Upon Tyne, Newcastle Upon Tyne, United Kingdom

DAVID J. MUZINA, MD, Director, Bipolar Disorders Clinical Research Unit, Department of Psychiatry and Psychology, The Cleveland Clinic Lerner College of Medicine of Case University, Cleveland, Ohio

I. JULIAN OSUJI, PhD, Post-Doctoral Fellow in Neuropsychology, Department of Psychiatry, The University of Texas Southwestern Medical Center at Dallas, Dallas, Texas

JENNIFER L. PAYNE, MD, Assistant Professor of Psychiatry, Department of Psychiatry and Behavioral Sciences, Johns Hopkins School of Medicine, Baltimore, Maryland

JAMES B. POTASH, MD, MPH, Assistant Professor of Psychiatry, Department of Psychiatry and Behavioral Sciences, Johns Hopkins School of Medicine, Baltimore, Maryland

JAN SCOTT, MD, FRCPsych, Professor of Psychological Treatments Research, Division of Psychological Medicine, Institute of Psychiatry, De Crespigny Park, Denmark Hill, London, UK

VIVEK SINGH, MD, Assistant Professor, Department of Psychiatry, The University of Texas Health Science Center at San Antonio, San Antonio, Texas

JAIR C. SOARES, MD, Associate Professor of Psychiatry and Radiology, Krus Endowed Chair in Psychiatry, and Chief, Division of Mood and Anxiety Disorders, University of Texas Health Science Center; and Chief, VA Psychiatry Research, South Texas Veterans Health Care System, Audie L. Murphy Division, San Antonio, Texas

E. VIETA, MD, PhD, Director, Bipolar Disorders Program, Hospital Clinic, IDIBAPS, University of Barcelona, Barcelona, Spain

LAKSHMI N. YATHAM, MBBS, FRCPC, Michael Smith Foundation Senior Scholar, Professor of Psychiatry, and Director, Mood Disorders Clinical Research Unit, University of British Columbia, Vancouver, British Columbia, Canada

A.H. YOUNG, MB, ChB, MPhil, PhD, FRCPsych, Professor of Psychiatry, University of Newcastle Upon Tyne, Newcastle upon Tyne, United Kingdom; University of Barcelona, Barcelona, Spain

CONTENTS

Clearly, efforts directed toward phenotyping neuropsychiatric disorders using such measures, in addition to other clinical, neuroimaging, neurophysiologic, and genotypic information, may yield important insights into the development, nature, and course of illness. It is hoped that this understanding will lead to better identification of individuals who may be prone to greater cognitive impairment or decline and those who might be more responsive to specific treatments.

FORTHCOMING ISSUES

RECENT ISSUES

THE CLINICS ARE NOW AVAILABLE ONLINE!

For more information about Clinics:
http://www.theclinics.com

ELSEVIER
SAUNDERS

Psychiatr Clin N Am
28 (2005) xiii–xiv

PSYCHIATRIC
CLINICS
OF NORTH AMERICA

Preface

Bipolar Disorder

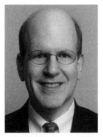

E. Sherwood Brown, MD, PhD
Guest Editor

It has been my great pleasure to serve as the Guest Editor for this issue of the *Psychiatric Clinics of North America*. Bipolar disorder is a common and disabling illness. Research on the cause and treatment of bipolar disorder has become one of the more active areas within psychiatry. I am very pleased that a number of outstanding scholars have contributed articles to this issue. The emphasis is on clinical aspects of bipolar disorder, although some recent basic science findings are also discussed.

In 2003 the editors of *Science* selected research on the genetics of psychiatric illnesses as a runner-up to breakthroughs in astronomy as the most outstanding scientific discovery of that year. The familial nature of bipolar disorder has long been appreciated, but recently a better understanding of the genetic underpinnings of the illness has evolved. Payne and DePaulo review recent findings on the ever-changing field of bipolar disorder genetics.

Our understanding of the mechanism of action of antidepressants and mood stabilizers has moved beyond explanations purely based on changes in neurotransmitter levels. Currently, neuroprotection and even neurogenesis are considered possible explanations of the efficacy of psychiatric medications. Lagace and Eisch discuss some of these important and clinically relevant findings in their article.

The remainder of the issue is devoted to clinical research, particularly treatment, although pertinent preclinical findings are frequently highlighted. The treatment armamentarium for bipolar disorder seems to grow each

0193-953X/05/$ - see front matter © 2005 Elsevier Inc. All rights reserved.
doi:10.1016/j.psc.2005.03.001   *psych.theclinics.com*

year. Antimanic agents now include not only lithium but numerous anti-seizure medications and atypical antipsychotics. Psychotherapy is also useful for many people who have bipolar disorder. The awareness that many people with bipolar disorder spend much more time depressed than manic has increased interest in the treatment of bipolar depression. Bipolar disorder can be a childhood illness. However, much minimal research has been conducted in children with bipolar disorder. Thus several articles on the treatment of adults and children with bipolar disorder are included in this issue.

Some of the many co-occurring conditions associated with bipolar disorder are also discussed. Perhaps the most common comorbidity of bipolar disorder is substance abuse. I have contributed an article on recent research in this area. Although perhaps less extensively studied than in schizophrenia, cognitive impairment is common in bipolar disorder. Osuji and Cullum review this topic. The neuroendocrine abnormalities associated with major depression, particularly hypothalamic–pituitary–adrenal axis activation, have been extensively described. These abnormalities are also very common in bipolar disorder. The article by Daban and colleagues covers this important topic. Functional, biochemical, and structural changes have been reported in the brains of people with bipolar disorder. Brambilla and collegues review bipolar disorder neuroimaging data.

I want to thank each of the authors who contributed articles to this issue. I also want to thank the authors of the work cited in the articles, because they provided the knowledge base that made these literature reviews possible. The field is changing rapidly, which is good news for both patients and physicians. I sincerely hope an updated issue on the topic of bipolar disorder will be required very soon, because this will be a yet another sign of the rapid progress being made in this area.

E. Sherwood Brown, MD, PhD
Assistant Professor and Director
Psychoneuroendocrine Research Program
Department of Psychiatry
University of Texas Southwestern Medical Center
5323 Harry Hines Boulevard
Dallas, TX 75390-8849, USA

E-mail address: sherwood.brown@utsouthwestern.edu

ELSEVIER
SAUNDERS

Psychiatr Clin N Am
28 (2005) 301–323

PSYCHIATRIC
CLINICS
OF NORTH AMERICA

Anticonvulsants in Bipolar Disorder

Vivek Singh, MD[a,*], David J. Muzina, MD[b],
Joseph R. Calabrese, MD[c,d]

[a]Department of Psychiatry, The University of Texas Health Science Center at San Antonio,
7703 Floyd Curl Drive (Mail Code 7792), San Antonio, TX 78229, USA
[b]Bipolar Disorders Clinical Research Unit, Department of Psychiatry and Psychology,
The Cleveland Clinic Lerner College of Medicine of Case University, 9500 Euclid Avenue,
P57, Cleveland OH 44195, USA
[c]Bipolar Disorder Research Center, Case University School of Medicine, Cleveland, OH, USA
[d]Mood Disorders Program, University Hospitals of Cleveland, 11400 Euclid Avenue,
Suite #200, Cleveland, OH 44106, USA

Bipolar disorder is a life-threatening illness that is complex and challenging to treat acutely and to manage long-term. The past decade has seen the emergence of anticonvulsants or antiepileptic drugs (AEDs) as viable and safe pharmacologic options in acute and long-term management of bipolar disorder. In addition, there has been a shift in focus from acute or episodic control of symptoms to the long-term management and prevention of further mood episodes that could worsen the course of illness.

The underlying pathophysiologic mechanisms in bipolar disorder are poorly understood. Evidence from preclinical studies suggests that bipolar disorder may share some biologic mechanisms with epilepsy. It has been hypothesized that an imbalance between the excitatory (primarily glutamate) and inhibitory (mainly γ-aminobutyric acid [GABA]) amino acids and dysfunctional cation pumps (sodium and calcium channels) may be involved in the pathogenesis of both epilepsy and bipolar disorder [1]. Bipolar disorder is characterized by recurrent episodes of mania or hypomania, either concomitantly or in alteration with a depressive episode. The characteristic episodic pattern of epileptic supports the hypothesis that bipolar disorder and epilepsy share a common pathophysiologic process. Earlier observations of the antimanic property of carbamazepine, an anticonvulsant, led to the proposal by Post and colleagues [2] that epilepsy and bipolar disorder could be conceptualized as sharing a common underlying biologic mechanism

---

* Corresponding author.
  E-mail address: singhv@uthscsa.edu (V. Singh).

called kindling. In kindling, repeated subthreshold neuronal stimulation generates an action potential sufficient to induce a seizure in epileptic patients and different mood states—mania, depression, or mixed states—in patients with bipolar disorder. It was then proposed that the progression of bipolar illness could be conceptualized by an animal model of kindled seizures and that this model could be used to screen antiepileptic drugs as candidate therapeutic agents for the treatment of bipolar illness [1]. Although this hypothesis was viewed at the time as scientifically appealing, it has never been confirmed or supported by empiric human clinical data.

This article reviews the role of the AEDs in the treatment of bipolar disorder with a special focus on data from randomized, placebo-controlled studies. It focuses on the role of valproate or divalproex sodium (DIV), carbamazepine (CBZ), oxcarbazepine (OXC), and lamotrigine (LAM) in the acute and long-term treatment of bipolar disorder and summarizes acute and longitudinal data on the newer anticonvulsants, gabapentin (GBP), topiramate (TMP), zonisamide (ZON), levetiracetam (LEV), and phenytoin (PHT), in bipolar disorder. It reviews the literature about the pharmacologic profiles (Table 1), safety, and tolerability of each of the AED.

Valproate or divalproex sodium

DIV has a potent action on the GABA system and, to a lesser extent, possesses antiglutamatergic properties [3]. Serendipitously, DIV was noted to possess behavioral effects in patients with bipolar disorder [4]. Following a large, confirmatory, randomized, double-blind, placebo parallel-group clinical trial of DIV versus lithium versus placebo in 1994, DIV was approved by the United States Food and Drug Administration (FDA) for the treatment of acute mania in 1995.

Acute efficacy

Acute mania
The antimanic efficacy of DIV has been compared in different studies to placebo, lithium, and haloperidol [5–8]. DIV demonstrated significant superiority to placebo (53% versus 10% response rates) in the first preliminary parallel-design, placebo-controlled study conducted by Pope et al [6]. Subsequently, Bowden and colleagues [7] conducted a large, three-arm study, comparing DIV to placebo, with lithium as the active comparator. The response rates in the DIV, lithium, and the placebo groups were 48%, 49%, and 25%, respectively. DIV demonstrated superior efficacy, compared with lithium, in a subset of patients with mixed mania [9] and in patients whose mania was associated with depressive symptoms [10]. This finding was also noted in another parallel-group study conducted by Freeman et al [11]. In the study by Bowden et al [7], which used an unbalanced study design, DIV also demonstrated better tolerability than lithium, and there

Table 1
Comparative pharmacologic profiles of anticonvulsants used in bipolar disorder

	DIV	CBZ	OXC	LAM	GBP	TMP	ZON	LEV	PHT
Time to steady state (d)	1–3	21–28[a]	2	3–15	1–2	4–5	5–15	2	7–28
Half-life (h)	9–16	12–17[b]	2–9[c]	25–30	5–7	19–23	63	6–8	7–22
Bioavailability (%)	>95	85	100	98	60–27[d]	80	100	100	100
Protein binding (%)	90–95	40–90	40	40–50	0–3	13–17	40	<10	93–98
Metabolism	Liver	Liver	Liver/biliary	Liver	None	Minimal	Liver	Liver	Liver
Clinically relevant metabolite	2-propyl-4-pentenoic acid (may cause toxicity)	10,11-epoxide (clinically active and may cause toxicity)	10-hydroxy carbazepine (clinically active)	None	None	None	None	None	None
Excretion	Renal	Renal	Renal	Renal	Renal	Renal	Renal	Renal	Renal
Dosage range (mg/d)	200–2500	200–1200	300–2400	50–400	600–3600	100–600	100–600	1000–3000	100–400
Target blood levels (μg/mL)	50–125	6–12	10–35	N	N	N	10–40	N	10–20
Monitoring of drug levels	R	R	NR	NR	NR	NR	N	NR	NR
Monitoring of liver functions	R	R	NR	NR	NR	R	NR	NR	NR
Monitoring of renal functions	NR	NR	NR	NR	NR	NR	NR	NR	NR
Monitoring of blood counts	R	R	NR	NR	NR	NR	NR	NR	NR
Monitoring of lipids	NR	NR	NR	NR	NR	NR	NR	NR	NR
Monitoring of blood sugar	NR	NR	NR	NR	NR	NR	NR	NR	NR
US-FDA pregnancy category	D	D	C	C	C	C	C	C	D

Abbreviations: CBZ, carbamazepine; C_{max}, time to peak plasma concentration; DIV, valproate or divalproex; GBP, gabapentin; LAM, lamotrigine; LEV, levetiracetam; N, not defined; NR, not required; OXC, oxcarbazepine; PHE, phenytoin or fosphenytoin; R, required; TMP, topiramate; ZON, zonisamide.

From Refs. [1,43,55,66].

[a] For completion of autoinduction.

[b] Because of autoinduction.

[c] 2 hours for parent compound, 9 hours for active metabolite.

[d] 60% at 900 mg/d in divided doses and progressively decreases to 27% at 4800 mg/d in divided doses.

were fewer dropouts in the DIV group than in the placebo group. DIV was similarly more efficacious than haloperidol in patients with psychotic mania [8] and to olanzapine in two studies [12,13].

DIV is effective when used in combination with other medications used in the treatment of mania, as demonstrated by several randomized, double-blind, placebo-controlled studies. Three of these studies, involving the addition of an antipsychotic drug to either DIV or lithium, demonstrated that the combination groups required lower doses of the antipsychotic drug in comparison to monotherapy with an antipsychotic [13–15]. The addition of DIV to haloperidol led to greater improvement in symptoms of mania than did haloperidol alone [16]. The response rate was similarly greater when either risperidone [14,15] or olanzapine [13] was added to DIV or lithium than when the mood stabilizers were continued as monotherapy. In the study by Sachs et al [14], patients enrolled had been either nonresponsive after receiving monotherapy with lithium or DIV at an adequate dose for 2 weeks or longer (add-on therapy group) or had been in a manic state without any treatment. In the latter group, treatment with risperidone and either lithium or valproate was initiated concomitantly (cotherapy group). Analysis of the data did not show any advantage for the combination treatment in the cotherapy group, but add-on therapy was advantageous in the group of patients who did not respond to DIV or lithium monotherapy. Each of the other studies required some degree of failure with monotherapy before addition of the second medication. Hence, these studies suggest that combination therapy is indicated in patients who have had no response or partial response to a short period of adequate treatment with a first anti-manic drug.

Bipolar depression

A small, blinded, randomized study demonstrated equivalent efficacy when DIV, paroxetine, or lithium was added to lithium (n = 19) or DIV (n = 8) in patients with bipolar depression. DIV was added to the regimen of patients taking lithium, lithium was added for patients taking DIV, and paroxetine was added to either lithium or DIV. The rate of discontinuation was lower in the group receiving paroxetine plus mood stabilizer than in the group taking DIV plus lithium [17,18]. A double-blind, parallel-group, placebo-controlled study (n = 45) to assess the efficacy of DIV in acute bipolar depression included subjects meeting *Diagnostic and Statistical Manual IV* criteria for bipolar disorder types I or II and criteria for a current major depressive episode [19]. This study included a 14-day, single-blind, placebo lead-in phase followed by an 8-week, double-blind, treatment phase and then an open-treatment phase of up to 8 weeks. Patients were considered recovered if there was absence of hypomania (Young Mania Rating Scale [YMRS] < 10) and an improvement of 50% or more on the 26-item Hamilton Depression Rating Scale (HDRS). Forty-three percent of the patients treated with DIV (9/21) met criteria for recovery compared with 27% of the patients treated with placebo (6/21). At every follow-up assessment, the patients treated with DIV demonstrated more improvement on the HAM-D depressed mood item than patients taking placebo, and this difference reached statistical significance at weeks 2, 4, and 5. Results from two other preliminary studies suggest that DIV is efficacious in the acute management of recurrent major depression and combat-related posttraumatic stress disorder [20,21].

DIV may have better efficacy in preventing depressive episodes or depressive symptoms during long-term treatment than in treating acute bipolar depression [18]. In a randomized, double-blind, parallel-group study over a 52-week maintenance period, bipolar type I patients were assigned to DIV, lithium, or placebo. The use of adjunctive sertraline or paroxetine was allowed for breakthrough depression. In the subgroup of patients taking the antidepressants, significantly more patients taking placebo than DIV discontinued treatment early because of depression. Patients taking DIV had less worsening of depressive symptoms than the subgroup of patients taking lithium, and they had a lower probability of relapse into depression, particularly if they had demonstrated a response to DIV when manic [22].

Maintenance efficacy

In a large, double-blind, placebo-controlled study [23], patients with bipolar disorder type I (n = 372) were randomly assigned to 1 year of maintenance treatment with DIV, lithium, or placebo after meeting recovery criteria within 3 months of an index manic episode. The time to develop any new full mood episode, the primary measure of efficacy, did not differ significantly among the treatment groups, although there was a trend of superiority for the DIV group. Secondary measures included time to a manic episode, time to a depressive episode, and Global Assessment of Function scores. The DIV group, when compared with placebo, had lower rates of early discontinuation for onset of any mood episode, onset of a depressive episode, and dropout for any reason [22,18]. DIV was superior to lithium in prolonging the duration of successful prophylaxis in the study, with less worsening of depressive symptomatology and Global Assessment of Function scores.

A separate 47-week maintenance study in bipolar patients with an index episode of acute mania found no significant differences between DIV and olanzapine in the rates of manic relapse or in the median time to a manic relapse [13].

Dosage and serum-level monitoring

Patients with serum levels greater than 45 µg/mL were significantly more likely to have at least 20% improvement in manic symptomatology than patients whose serum level was lower than 45 µg/mL [18,24]. During maintenance treatment, valproate levels between 75 and 100 µg/mL were more likely to maintain prophylaxis than serum levels higher or lower than this range. Another study showed that adjustments of DIV dosing based on serum valproate levels were associated with a reduction in length of hospital stay [25].

Tolerability

DIV is well tolerated, as evidenced in the largest maintenance trial with DIV, in which reported weight gain and tremors were the only symptoms seen more commonly with DIV than with placebo [23]. Common dose- or serum level–related side effects seen with DIV include tremors (9% to 22%) [26], sedation (24%) [26], reduction in platelets (1%–32%) [27] and white blood cell count (0.4%) [27], nausea (22%), vomiting (14%), and alopecia (2%–22%). Extremely low rates of hepatotoxicity (1/49,000) and pancreatitis (<1%), which are idiosyncratic in nature and more commonly seen in younger patients, do not justify the routine monitoring of hepatic function and amylase levels. DIV is FDA pregnancy category D and has been associated with neural tube defects (1%–4%) [18].

Carbamazepine

CBZ has been hypothesized to reduce kindling, enhances GABAergic transmission, and has antiglutamatergic properties in addition to its cellular and intracellular actions [3]. It was the first AED widely used in the treatment of bipolar disorder.

Acute efficacy

Acute mania

Sixteen controlled trials have been conducted to assess the efficacy of CBZ in acute mania, but the interpretation of the results of many of these studies is difficult. Early trials were limited by the absence of a parallel placebo group, small sample sizes, and the use of other antimanic drugs during the study [28–30]. Recently, in the first large, randomized, double-blind, placebo-controlled trial using extended-release CBZ capsules (ERC-CBZ) in acute mania, ERC-CBZ demonstrated superior efficacy to placebo (response rate 41.5% versus 22.4%) with significant improvement in mixed manic patients. In addition to demonstrating ERC-CBZ's efficacy, the study showed that it is well tolerated. Pooled data from five randomized, double-blind, controlled trials of CBZ in acute mania have demonstrated equivalent responses with CBZ, lithium, and chlorpromazine (50%, 56%, and 68% respectively) [29].

Bipolar depression

Although a moderate antidepressant effect was seen in a placebo-controlled trial of CBZ monotherapy, this study was limited by its small sample size (n = 13) and the inclusion of patients with diagnosis of schizoaffective disorder, bipolar type and unipolar depression in addition to patients with bipolar disorder [31,32]. In a study of 35 patients with bipolar depression, Post and colleagues [33] reported that 57% experienced mild improvement, and 34% marked improvement (average dose, 971 mg/day). These preliminary data suggest that CBZ may possess some acute antidepressant efficacy, but more rigorously controlled investigation of its antidepressant efficacy is needed.

Maintenance efficacy

There is a paucity of data on the efficacy of CBZ in long-term management of bipolar illness [34]. In the only placebo-controlled study to assess the maintenance effectiveness of CBZ in bipolar disorder, CBZ demonstrated significant superiority to placebo [35]. An open-label, 2.5-year, randomized maintenance study found lithium to be superior to CBZ using broader efficacy measures that included time to relapse, time to receiving additional medications, or intolerance. There was no difference between the two groups on the primary efficacy measure, time to rehospitalization for a new mood episode. CBZ demonstrated superior efficacy in patients with atypical forms of mania [36,37]. When functional improvement is used as a measure, a combination of lithium and CBZ is more effective than either agent used as monotherapy [38].

Dosage and serum-level monitoring

Because of CBZ's induction of its metabolism and the associated adverse events relating to the central nervous system, particularly in the early course of treatment, CBZ should be started at low doses (100–400 mg/day) and increased gradually until response or adverse events ensue or serum levels exceed 12 µg/mL [3]. Correlation between serum level and response to CBZ has not been established in bipolar disorder.

Tolerability

The acute and long-term utility of CBZ is limited significantly by its side-effect profile. The discontinuation rate because of adverse events in a randomized, double-blind, crossover maintenance study was higher in the CBZ group (22%) than in the lithium group (4%) [38]. Dose-related adverse effects with CBZ include dizziness, sedation, ataxia, diplopia, and nystagmus, all of which are reversible [28]. CBZ is associated with a mild rash in 10% of the patients, which may be the harbinger of a life-threatening Stevens-Johnson syndrome. Agranulocytosis and aplastic anemia, idiosyncratic in nature, occur in 1/10,000 to 1/100,000 patients; benign leukopenia (transient in 10% of patients and persistent in 2%) is more common. Thrombocytopenia occurs in 2% of patients treated with CBZ. CBZ may also cause mild hyponatremia, which may manifest more seriously in geriatric or medically ill patients. The side effects associated with CBZ are attributed to its major metabolite, CBZ-(10;11)-epoxide.

CBZ, by its induction of the cytochrome P450 enzymes, particularly P450-3A4, causes lowering of plasma levels of other drugs such as anticonvulsants (DIV, LAM, ZON, TMP, CBZ, PHT, OXC, and others) antipsychotics (aripiprazole, clozapine, haloperidol, olanzapine, risperidone, ziprasidone, and others), antidepressants (bupropion, citalopram, tricyclic antidepressants), anxiolytics/sedatives (buspirone, clonazepam, alprazolam, and others), stimulants (methylphenidate, modafinil) and oral contraceptives [28,39]. To maintain their continual efficacy, higher doses of medications such as oral contraceptives must be used when they are taken concomitantly with CBZ.

CBZ's limited clinical utility and its role as an alternative rather than a first-line treatment option in bipolar illness can be attributed to its propensity to cause drug–drug interactions, its FDA pregnancy category D drug classification, and lack of an FDA indication in bipolar disorder [28].

Oxcarbazepine

OXC is a 10-keto derivative of CBZ, and it is hypothesized that its structural similarity to CBZ bestows on it similar mechanistic actions [28] and similar effects in bipolar disorder. It is free of some of the side-effect and drug–drug limitations associated with CBZ. It is postulated that OXC's efficacy in bipolar illness results from its ability to block voltage-sensitive Na^+ and to modulate voltage-activated Ca^{++} currents [39].

Acute efficacy

Acute mania

Two blinded studies, each lasting 15 days, comparing OXC with active comparators lithium and haloperidol, demonstrated equivalent efficacy in the treatment of acute mania [39,40]. In the first study comparing OXC (n = 17) with haloperidol (n = 20), 16 of 17 patients receiving OXC showed improvement, whereas improvement was seen in 15 of 20 patients taking haloperidol. OXC was superior to haloperidol in tolerability (rate of adverse events, 10% versus 35%). In a comparison with lithium, 27 of 29 patients taking OXC showed improvement, whereas 22 of 24 patients taking lithium improved. Small sample sizes and the absence of a placebo group limit conclusions from these studies.

Bipolar depression

No studies have been conducted to date to asses the efficacy of OXC in bipolar depression, although OXC's efficacy in two animal models of depression, learned helplessness and forced swimming [39], suggest efficacy in depression.

Maintenance efficacy

There is a lack of direct evidence for OXC in the long-term management of bipolar disorder, with only 12 patients enrolled in long-term studies using OXC [28]. Given the similarities in mechanism of action between CBZ and OXC, it may be hypothesized that CBZ and OXC have similar spectra of activity in bipolar disorder.

Dosage and serum-level monitoring

The doses for OXC are about 50% higher than doses for CBZ, and it is usually dosed between 900 to 2400 mg/day. The serum concentration for OXC recommended for treatment in epilepsy is usually between 10 and 35 μg/mL. As with CBZ, the dose of OXC should be titrated until response is attained or adverse events ensue, with the serum-concentration range used as guide, particularly in regards to pharmacologic safety.

Tolerability

OXC has therapeutic and adverse effects similar to CBZ [28] but is better tolerated than CBZ, perhaps because of its minimal protein-binding property and the absence of the active epoxide metabolite [41]. OXC has a lower propensity to cause leukopenia, agranulocytosis, rash, induction of its own metabolism, and drug–drug interaction [2,39,42]. Averse events commonly seen with OXC include somnolence, dizziness, diplopia, nausea, and ataxia [43]. Because OXC does not cause aplastic anemia and agranulocytosis, hematologic monitoring is not warranted. OXC has a higher incidence of hyponatremia (2.5%) than CBZ, and about 25% to 30% of patients with a hypersensitivity to CBZ experience a reaction to OXC [39,44]. OXC, like CBZ, lowers plasma levels of oral contraceptives, necessitating higher doses of contraceptives or use of alternative contraception for continued protection from pregnancy. OXC is a FDA pregnancy category C drug.

Lamotrigine

LAM inhibits the flux of sodium at use-dependent and voltage-sensitive N^+ channels and has antiglutamatergic action, which may explain its efficacy in the treatment of bipolar disorder. Anecdotal reports of its beneficial effects on mood during its development as an anticonvulsant led to investigation of its usefulness in the treatment of bipolar disorder.

Acute efficacy

Acute mania

LAM has been shown not to possess efficacy in the treatment of acute mania [45,46] and is not recommended as either monotherapy or as an adjunct to another antimanic agent in this mood state.

Bipolar depression

One large-scale, placebo-controlled trial has demonstrated LAM's efficacy in the acute treatment of bipolar depression. One hundred ninety-five bipolar I patients meeting criteria for a major depressive episode were randomly assigned to treatment with LAM (50 mg/day), LAM (200 mg/day), or placebo in a 7-week, multicenter, double-blinded, placebo-controlled study conducted by Calabrese et al [47]. Patients in the LAM, 200 mg/day, group had a significant improvement in depressive symptomatology as measured by the Montgomery-Asberg Depression Rating Scale, HAM-D 17, CGI-Severity scale, and CG I-Improvement scale as compared with placebo. Improvement was seen as early as week 3 in both the active treatment groups compared with placebo. On several measures, the efficacy of LAM, 50 mg, was similar to placebo. No significant differences in the rates of switch into mania, hypomania, or a mixed state were observed between the LAM and placebo groups (4.6%–5.4% versus 5%) without concomitant medications. In a second randomized, 6-week, placebo-controlled trial [48] using a crossover design in treatment-refractory bipolar (n = 25) and unipolar (n = 6) patients, a significantly greater number of patients had substantial reduction in depressive symptomatology with LAM than with placebo (45% versus 19%). Secondary analysis of these data with an expanded cohort (n = 45) revealed that response to LAM was associated a diagnosis of bipolar disorder, fewer prior hospitalizations, fewer previous medication trials, and male gender.

The studies discussed here demonstrate acute efficacy of LAM in the treatment of bipolar depression, the most common mood state in this illness. In addition, LAM may be a safer alternative to antidepressants, as long as patients do not develop serious rashes, because it does not cause cycle acceleration, mixed states, or switching to mania or hypomania, which worsen long-term prognosis.

Maintenance efficacy

LAM was the second agent approved by the FDA for maintenance treatment in bipolar disorder. This approval followed two paired, randomized, parallel-group, placebo-controlled, multicenter studies that demonstrated its efficacy in maintenance treatment in patients with bipolar I disorder [49,50]. The two studies were designed to assess the efficacy and tolerability of LAM and lithium compared with placebo for preventing relapse or recurrence of any mood episode in bipolar I patients. Both studies consisted of a screening phase of up to 2 weeks; an open-label phase of to 8 to 16 weeks during which treatment with LAM (100–200 mg/day) was started as monotherapy or adjunctive treatment and other psychotropic agents were gradually tapered off; and an 18-month double-blind phase during which patients were randomly assigned to LAM (100–400 mg/day), lithium (flexibly dosed to achieve blood levels of 0.8–1.1 mEq/L), or placebo. The first study included patients with a recent episode of mania or hypomania (n = 175) [49]. The second study included patients with a recent major depressive episode (n = 463) [50]. The primary efficacy measure in both the studies was time to intervention for any mood episode. In both studies, both LAM and lithium were superior to placebo. In addition, in both studies, LAM, but not lithium, was superior to placebo in delaying relapse in depression; the opposite was true for delaying time to relapse in mania. In a planned, pooled combined analysis of the two studies, both LAM and lithium were significantly more efficacious than placebo on the primary efficacy measure, time to intervention for any mood episode. Whereas LAM, but not lithium, demonstrated superiority to placebo in prolonging time to a depressive episode, both LAM and lithium were more efficacious than placebo in prolonging time to a manic, hypomanic, or a mixed episode. Patients taking LAM had a higher risk of a recurrence or relapse to an episode of the same polarity than of an opposite one [51]. There was no difference between LAM and placebo in the rate of switching to mania, hypomania, or mixed states (5% versus 7%).

In a large, 26-week, placebo-controlled trial in patients with rapid cycling subtype of bipolar disorder (n = 182), LAM (100–500 mg/day) did not separate from placebo in the primary outcome measure, time to intervention with additional pharmacotherapy for an emerging mood episode, in the general cohort of patients and in those with bipolar I disorder but showed a trend toward superiority in patients with bipolar II disorder [52]. Survival analysis (time to dropout for any reason) demonstrated LAM's superiority over placebo in the general cohort of patients and in those with bipolar II disorder but showed no significant separation from placebo in bipolar I patients. This study provides evidence for the role of LAM in rapid cycling subtype of bipolar disorder, particularly in bipolar II patients.

Dosing

LAM should be gradually titrated to minimize the probability of emergence of adverse events, particularly a serious rash. The recommended titration is: 25 mg/day for the first 2 weeks, then 50 mg/day for weeks 3 and 4, and then increasing by 50 to 100 mg/week to 200 mg/day or as clinically indicated [53]. If LAM is part of a combination regimen involving CBZ, an inducer of LAM's metabolism, the starting dose of LAM should be doubled, and the titration should be more rapid. On the other hand, in a combination regimen involving DIV, the starting dose of LAM should be halved, and titration slowed, because DIV inhibits the metabolism of LAM (Table 2).

Tolerability

LAM is well tolerated and in placebo-controlled trials seems to be devoid of the polarity switches or cycle acceleration seen with antidepressants [50]. Headache, ataxia, dizziness, tremors, nausea, somnolence, diplopia, and blurred vision are the most common side effects reported with LAM [2,41–43]. LAM does not negatively affect weight, cognition, or sexual functioning [50]. In a published analysis of the rates of rash in 12 multicenter clinical trials involving 3153 patients exposed to LAM, 11.6% developed a benign rash, and less than 0.1% developed a serious rash [50]. Oral contraceptives (ethinylestradiol and levonorgestrel), when administered with LAM in an open-label, non–placebo-controlled study (n = 22), caused a significant decrease in serum levels of LAM (area under the curve by 52%; time to reach peak concentration by 39%) during the 21 days that the oral contraceptives where taken. By the end of the pill-free period, the trough concentration of LAM had increased by two times [53]. This interaction may decrease the efficacy of LAM when the use of oral contraceptives is initiated in a patient taking a steady dose of LAM. It may also increase the risk of rash during the pill-free period. The FDA originally described LAM as a pregnancy category C drug. The 2005 Interim Report of the International Lamotrigine Pregnancy Registry, however, reported data on the teratogenic potential of LAM based on the observed frequency of birth defects in patients with first trimester exposure to LAM monotherapy, which was 2.9% (95% confidence interval [CI], 1.6–4.9) compared with a background rate estimated at 2% to 3% [54]. The rate of birth defects among patients exposed to LAM and valproate cotherapy during the first trimester was 11.9% (95% CI, 6.6–20.2), compared with a rate of 2.9% (05% CI, 1.2–6.5) for patients receiving LAM polytherapy that did not

Table 2
Dosing of lamotrigine

	LAM alone	LAM + DIV	LAM + CBZ
Weeks 1 and 2	25 mg/d	25 mg every other day	25 mg two ×/d
Weeks 3 and 4	50 mg/d	25 mg/d	50 mg two ×/d
Week 5	100 mg/d	50 mg/d	100 mg two ×/d
Week 6	200 mg/d	100 mg/d	150 mg two ×/d
Week 7			200 mg two ×/d

Abbreviations: CBZ, carbamazepine; DIV, valproate or divalproex; LAM, lamotrigine.

include valproate as part of the treatment regimen. These preliminary data suggest that the rates of teratogenicity secondary to LAM exposure during the first trimester of pregnancy (2.9%) are similar to background rates in the epilepsy population (2%–3%) [54].

Topiramate

The mechanism by which TMP exerts its efficacy in epilepsy is not well understood. It affects the voltage-dependent sodium channels and GABA receptors and acts as an antagonist at the glutamate receptor. These varied actions may be responsible for its antiepileptic property, its potential effectiveness in bipolar illness, and possibly its action in substance abuse and eating disorders [3,55,56].

Acute efficacy

Acute mania

TMP has no efficacy, as a monotherapeutic agent in the treatment of acute mania, as demonstrated by five double-blind, placebo-controlled trials [56]. Some open-label studies and case reports have suggested a role for TMP in the treatment of acute mania, but its use in the treatment of acute mania is not recommended because it is not supported by the preponderance of controlled data.

Bipolar depression

An open-label study (n = 45) indicated that TMP (100–400 mg/day) may have some efficacy in the treatment of bipolar depression [1]. Nineteen of the 31 patients completing the study responded well to TMP, whereas 12 showed a partial response as measured by the HDRS. In a single-blind (rater blinded), randomized study, 36 currently depressed bipolar patients were assigned to receive either bupropion (50–300 mg/day) or TMP (100–400 mg/day) in addition lithium or DIV. TMP (56%) and bupropion (59%) demonstrated equivalent efficacy, based on a prior-response criterion of a 50% reduction on the HDRS [57]. Both TMP and bupropion were well tolerated, but patients taking TMP had greater weight loss than patients on bupropion.

TMP is associated with weight loss in psychiatric patients and in those with epilepsy. In a double-blind study involving patients with binge-eating disorder (n = 61), TMP (mean dose, 212 g/day) caused a significantly larger decrease in the frequency of binging and weight [3,56]. These data are promising, given the propensity of medications used in bipolar disorder to cause significant weight gain. TMP may play a critical role as an adjunct to a first-line mood stabilizer in minimizing weight gain associated with the primary mood stabilizers.

314 SINGH et al

Maintenance efficacy

One large, open-label study (n = 58) has been conducted to assess the efficacy of TMP in the long-term management of bipolar disorder [58]. Patients with an index episode of mania received both TMP and risperidone. Risperidone could be discontinued at any point, but patients had to take TMP for 12 months to be considered study completers. Seventy-one percent of the patients completed the study. Substantial improvement was noted on the YMRS and the CGI-Bipolar Disorder scales. The rates of relapse during the 12 months of the study were lower than the rates seen in the previous year. Because of the lack of data from controlled trials, however, TMP should not be considered a primary option in the long-term management of bipolar disorder.

Dosing

Treatment with TMP should be started at 25 mg/day and titrated up by 25 mg every 4 to 7 days to a dosage range of 100 to 400 mg/day to minimize adverse events and enhance compliance.

Tolerability

Headache (32%), dizziness (24%), anxiety (24%), and dyspepsia (18%) were the most commonly reported adverse events in the controlled study in acute mania. Other common side effects seen with TMP are paresthesias, anorexia, nausea, diarrhea, headache, fatigue, and somnolence [1,55]. Cognitive difficulties and psychomotor slowing common and may be the limiting factors in either the use of TMP or its use at higher dose ranges. Nephrolithiasis occurs in 1% of the patients treated with TMP, with risk escalation associated with use of other carbonic anhydrase inhibitors such as acetazolamide and zonisamide [3]. TMP has not been associated with congenital malformations in humans (FDA pregnancy category C).

Gabapentin

GBP was developed as an analogue of GABA, the major inhibitory neurotransmitter in the human brain. It seems to bind to an amino acid transporter and acts at a unique receptor [55]. GBP does not act as a GABA precursor, agonist, or antagonist but increases the GABA levels in the brain and intracellularly by various mechanisms [59]. It also possesses a modulatory action on voltage-sensitive calcium channels [55]. Its low side-effect profile, coupled with its lack of drug–drug interaction and safety at high doses, make it a safe option in the treatment of bipolar disorder. Its use as a first-line agent in the treatment of acute and long-term bipolar illness, however, is limited by the lack of data from controlled studies.

Acute efficacy

Acute mania

The efficacy of GBP (600–3600 mg/day, flexible dosing) as add-on therapy to lithium or DIV was evaluated in a double-blind, placebo-controlled study with bipolar I patients (n = 117) in manic, hypomanic, or mixed states [60]. In the first phase of the study lasting 2 weeks, single-blind, flexible dosing of GBP was used versus single-blind placebo lead-in. This first phase was followed by 10-week, double-blind phase during which patients were randomly assigned to either GBP or placebo. Placebo demonstrated superiority over GBP on the primary efficacy measure, total decrease on the YMRS. The results of the study might have been confounded by non-compliance (20% of patients on GBP had undetectable plasma levels of the drug) and high rates of placebo response because of the larger proportion of lithium-dosage adjustment in patients taking placebo (75%, 9/12).

In another double-blind, placebo-controlled, crossover study comparing the efficacy of GBP monotherapy (up to 4800 mg/day), LAM (up to 500 mg/day), and placebo in treatment-refractory mood disorder in 35 in-patients for 6 weeks, GBP did not separate from placebo [59]. Of the patients who responded to GBP, response was associated with younger age, shorter duration of illness, and lower baseline weight.

Recommendation of GBP as an agent of choice or even as a first-line alternative in either acute mania or depression is not justified because of the lack of efficacy seen in controlled trials. Because of its anxiolytic properties [60,61], however, GBP may be used as an adjunct to first-line mood stabilizers in bipolar patients with comorbid anxiety disorders.

Maintenance efficacy

There is a paucity data from controlled trials assessing the efficacy of GBP in maintenance treatment of bipolar disorder. The use of GBP, as monotherapy in the long-term treatment of bipolar disorder is not recommended.

Dosing

GBP has a nonlinear bioavailability because the amino acid transporter responsible for its absorption in the gut and its transport through the blood–brain barrier is saturable. Plasma concentrations of GBP plateau at single doses higher than 1200 mg, three times a day. Treatment with GBP should be started at 300 mg/day and titrated to 900 mg/day within 3 days. GBP must be administered in three-times-per-day dosing [55].

Tolerability

GBP is generally well tolerated, has no active metabolite, and has minimal drug–drug interactions [59]. Common adverse events reported include sedation, dizziness, drowsiness, ataxia, and dry mouth. GBP has an FDA pregnancy category C rating.

Zonisamide

ZON, an anticonvulsant with a structure similar to serotonin and a pharmacologic profile similar to CBZ, is thought to regulate the balance between inhibitory and excitatory amino acids in the brain by increasing the levels of GABA and by its antiglutamatergic properties [3,62]. Its blockade of voltage-sensitive sodium channels and reduction of voltage-dependent calcium channels may also play a role in its potential efficacy in bipolar illness [55]. ZON possesses weight-loss and sedative properties, characteristics that are seen in TMP as well.

Acute efficacy

Data from controlled studies evaluating the efficacy of ZON in acute mania or bipolar depression are lacking. An open-label study conducted in 1994 in 24 patients (15 with bipolar mania, 6 with schizoaffective mania, and 3 with schizophrenic excitement) demonstrated encouraging results, particularly in patients with bipolar mania [62]. It would be premature to conclude unequivocally that ZON is efficacious in acute mania because of the lack of evidence from rigorously controlled studies.

The most exciting aspect of ZON is its positive effect on weight. In a recent 16-week, double-blind, placebo-controlled study, ZON was significantly superior to placebo in causing mean weight loss (5.9 kg versus 0.9 kg) in obese nonpsychiatric adults. The superiority of ZON was even more substantial (9.2 kg versus 1.5 kg) when the study was continued in a single-blind extension for another 16 weeks [3,63]. These results are promising, because most drugs used in management of bipolar disorder (eg, the antipsychotics) cause weight gain, which negatively affects compliance. Given the ability of ZON to cause weight loss, it may have a role as an adjunct to other mood stabilizers when weight gain becomes the limiting factor in treatment compliance.

Dosing

ZON should not be administered to patients with allergy to sulfonamides, because ZON is a sulfonamide. Treatment with ZON is usually initiated at 100 mg/day and gradually increased by 100 mg every 2 weeks for a target dose of 100 to 600 mg/day [55].

Tolerability

The most commonly encountered side effects with ZON include sedation, dizziness, cognitive impairment, and nausea. These adverse events are concentration and dose dependent and hence improve with dose reduction [55]. Renal calculi occur in about 1% of patients, and the risk may increase if ZON is administered in combination with other carbonic anhydrase inhibitors such as acetazolamide and TMP. CBZ, an enzyme inducer, decreases the serum level of ZON. ZON has not been reported to cause congenital malformations in humans (FDA pregnancy category C).

Levetiracetam

LEV is a novel anticonvulsant with a broad spectrum of efficacy in epilepsy. Its antikindling and neuroprotective properties make it an attractive option for treatment of patients with bipolar disorder. Its efficacy is thought to result from its effect on the GABA system [3,64].

There has been a case report of efficacy of LEV in bipolar disorder, and an open, add-on study with 10 patients showed LEV to exhibit antimanic properties [65]. Controlled studies are needed to investigate the role of LEV in the treatment of bipolar disorder.

Dosing

Treatment with LEV is initiated at 1000 mg/day in two divided doses, increasing by 1000-mg increments every 2 weeks to a maximum recommended dose of 3000 mg/day (1500 mg twice a day).

Tolerability

LEV is generally well tolerated. The most commonly encountered adverse events include sedation, fatigue, lack of coordination, and a decline in red blood and white blood cells. To minimize dose-dependent adverse events and to enhance compliance, treatment with LEV may be initiated at half the rate and titrated more gradually. LEV is not associated with congenital malformations in humans (FDA pregnancy category C).

Phenytoin

Like many other antimanic anticonvulsants, PHT blocks voltage-activated sodium channels limiting the spread of seizure activity and seizure propagation. This action may suggest a therapeutic role for PHT in the management of bipolar disorder.

Acute efficacy

Only limited and inconsistent evidence suggests a potential role for PHT in the acute management of bipolar mania despite early reports by Kalinowsky and Putnam [67] that PHT was markedly beneficial for acute mania. Mishory and colleagues [68] reported a 5-week, double-blind, controlled trial of haloperidol plus PHT versus haloperidol plus placebo in 39 patients with either bipolar mania or schizoaffective mania. Significantly greater improvement was observed in the patients receiving PHT. Of note, additional improvements in scores on the Brief Psychiatric Rating Scale and CGI were seen in PHT-treated bipolar patients but not in the schizoaffective patients [68]. In a smaller sample of seven patients with mania, however, the intravenous administration of fosphenytoin (prodrug of PHT) did not produce any antimanic effects in any of the subjects during the 60 minutes of observation [69]. The dosing for fosphenytoin in this study is known to treat status epilepticus effectively, demonstrating its rapid onset of major neurobiologic effects, but it did not produce any beneficial effects for mania.

There are no data to support the use of PHT in the treatment of acute bipolar depression.

Maintenance efficacy

There is no evidence supporting PHT monotherapy for the prevention of mood episodes associated with bipolar disorder. Mishory and colleagues have reported a double-blind, placebo crossover study of PHT added to the ongoing mood stabilizing medication regimens of patients with bipolar disorder who had experienced at least one mood episode per year in the previous 2 years (Mishory et al, unpublished data). A significant prophylactic effect was observed with the addition of PHT, indicating a potential role for PHT as an add-on agent in patients with breakthrough mood episodes despite ongoing maintenance treatment with other agents. Replication of this study with a larger sample size is needed before acceptance of PHT's role in the long-term management of bipolar illness and to determine whether it possesses preferential prophylactic efficacy against the depressive or manic state of the illness.

Dosing

PHT should be avoided in individuals with a history of hypersensitivity to it or to other hydantoins. The dosing used in the Mishory et al study [64] (PHT, 100 mg/day as an add-on to other maintenance therapy) can be considered with 100-mg/day incremental increases each week to a target dose of 300 to 400 mg/day. Although a specific therapeutic blood range for bipolar disorder is not known, a potential target range of 10 to 20 µg/mL may be reasonable and is in line with the therapeutic blood range for epilepsy management and the blood levels observed by Mishory and colleagues.

Tolerability

The most common dose-dependent side effects reported with PHT therapy involve the central nervous system and include sedation, nystagmus, fatigue, slurred speech, ataxia, coordination difficulty, confusion, dizziness, and headaches [55]. Rashes, including a risk for Stevens-Johnson syndrome, have been encountered. Hemopoietic complications of all varieties, with or without bone marrow suppression, have occurred and may be fatal. Nausea, vomiting, constipation, arthralgias, and gingival hyperplasia are less serious, although common, complications of PHT treatment and may cause discomfort for some patients.

Summary

In recent years, a number of anticonvulsants have been more rigorously investigated for their potential mood-stabilizing properties. They are heterogeneous in their mechanisms of action and in their efficacy in the various mood states in bipolar illness (Table 3).

At present, evidence from well-controlled studies supports the role of DIV and CBZ in the treatment of acute mania. DIV seems to have better efficacy than lithium in mixed mania or mania associated with depressive symptoms and is recommended as a first-line pharmacologic option in acutely manic or mixed manic patients [10]. Neither CBZ nor DIV have robust evidence supporting their efficacy in the treatment of acute bipolar depression, although DIV clearly possesses beneficial effects on depressive symptomatology and prophylaxis against depressive episodes during long-term treatment. Results from a large study indicate that LAM has significant efficacy in bipolar depression without the associated risks of cycle acceleration or manic/hypomanic switches. LAM should be considered a primary option in patients with bipolar depression and in bipolar II

Table 3
Comparative efficacy of anticonvulsants in bipolar disorder[a]

	DIV	CBZ	OXC	LAM	GBP	TMP	ZON	LEV	PHT
Classic mania	+++	+++	+	−	−	−	−	−	+/−
Mixed mania	+++	++	−	−	−	−	−	−	−
Bipolar depression	+	+	−	++	−	+	−	−	−
Rapid cycling, bipolar disorder I	++	+/−	−	+	−	−	−	−	−
Rapid cycling, bipolar disorder II	+	+/−	−	++	−	−	−	−	−
Prophylaxis	++	+	−	+++	−	+/−	−	−	+/−

Abbreviations: CBZ, carbamazepine; DIV, valproate or divalproex; GBP, gabapentin; LAM, lamotrigine; LEV, levetiracetam; OXC, oxcarbazepine; PHE, phenytoin or fosphenytoin; TMP, topiramate; ZON, zonisamide.

Symbols: +, limited controlled data supporting efficacy; ++, controlled data supporting efficacy; +++, replicated, controlled data supporting efficacy; +/−, small studies with controlled data supporting efficacy; −, no data or data does not support efficacy.

[a] Based on amount and strength of controlled data; scored relative to other anticonvulsants only.

patients with rapid cycling. DIV is recommended as a first-line option in bipolar I patients with rapid cycling.

LAM has proven efficacy in the prophylaxis of bipolar I disorder and should be considered along with lithium or DIV as treatment of choice in the long-term management of bipolar disorder. For the other anticonvulsants, including CBZ and OXC, there is still inadequate evidence of efficacy as monotherapy in the long-term management of bipolar disorder. Even less data exist for other available AEDs, and consensus is growing that some AEDs (eg, GBP) have little or no specific effect in bipolar disorder.

Despite the progress made in the past decade, a wider therapeutic armamentarium is critically needed, because a large proportion of bipolar patients do not respond to acute treatments during a manic or depressive episode and have frequent relapse and recurrences during long-term treatment. As additional AEDs become available, rigorously designed and large-scale studies examining AEDs as monotherapy and AEDs in combination therapies versus placebo must be undertaken to assess efficacy and safety more adequately to provide better guidance for the clinician faced with the management of this challenging mood disorder.

References

[1] Chengappa KN, Gerhson S, Levine J. The evolving role of topiramate among other mood stabilizers in the management of bipolar disorder. Bipolar Disord 2001;3(5):215–32.
[2] Post RM, Uhde TW. Treatment of mood disorder with antiepileptic medications: clinical and theoretical implications. Epilepsia 1983;2:S97–108.
[3] Wang PW, Ketter TA, Becker OV, et al. New anticonvulsant medication uses in bipolar disorder. CNS Spectr 2003;(12):941–7.
[4] Lambert PA, Cavaz G, Borselli S, et al. Action neuropsychotrope d'un nouvel antiepileplique: le depamide. Ann Med Psychol 1966;1:707–10.
[5] Emrich HM, von Zerssen DKW, Moller HJ. On a possible role of GABA in mania: therapeutic efficacy of sodium valproate. Adv Biochem Psychopharmacol 1981;26:287–96.
[6] Pope HG Jr, McElroy SL, Keck PE Jr, et al. Valproate in the treatment of acute mania: a placebo-controlled study. Arch Gen Psychiatry 1991;48:62–8.
[7] Bowden CL. Efficacy of divalproex vs lithium and placebo in mania. JAMA 1994;272: 1005–6.
[8] McElroy PE, Keck SL, Tugrul KC, et al. Valproate as a loading treatment in acute mania. Neuropsychobiology 1993;27:146–9.
[9] Bowden CL, Calabrese JR, Wallin BA, et al. Illness characteristics of patients in clinical drug studies of mania. Psychopharmacol Bull 1995;31(1):103–9.
[10] Swann AC, Bowden CL, Morris D, et al. Depression during mania: treatment response to lithium or divalproex. Arch Gen Psychiatry 1997;54:37–42.
[11] Freeman TW, Clothier JL, Pazzaglia P, et al. A double-blind comparison of valproate and lithium in the treatment of acute mania. Am J Psychiatry 1992;149:108–11.
[12] Zajecka JM, Weisler R, Sachs G, et al. A comparison of the efficacy, safety, and tolerability of divalproex sodium and olanzapine in the treatment of bipolar disorder. J Clin Psychiatry 2002;63(12):1148–55.

[13] Tohen M, Ketter TA, Zarate CA. Olanzapine versus divalproex sodium for the treatment of acute mania and maintenance of remission: a 47-week study. Am J Psychiatry 2003;160: 1263–71.

[14] Sachs G, Grossman F, Okamoto A, et al. Risperidone plus mood stabilizer versus placebo plus mood stabilizer for acute mania of bipolar disorder: a double-blind comparison of efficacy and safety. Am J Psychiatry 2002;159:1146–54.

[15] Yatham LN, Grossman F, Augustyns I, et al. Mood stabilisers plus risperidone or placebo in the treatment of acute mania. International, double-blind, randomised controlled trial. Br J Psychiatry 2003;182:141–7.

[16] Muller-Oerlinghausen B, Retzow A, Henn FA, et al. Valproate as an adjunct to neuroleptic medication for the treatment of acute episodes of mania: a prospective, randomized, double-blind, placebo-controlled, multicenter study. J Clin Psychopharmacol 2000;20(2):195–203.

[17] Young LT, Joffe RT, Robb JC, et al. Double-blind comparison of addition of a second mood stabilizer versus an antidepressant to an initial mood stabilizer for treatment of patients with bipolar depression. Am J Psychiatry 2000;157(1):124–6.

[18] Bowden CL. Valproate. Bipolar Disord 2003;5(3):189–202.

[19] Sachs G, Altshuler L, Ketter T, et al. Divalproex versus placebo for the treatment of bipolar depression. Presented at the 40th Annual Meeting of the American College of Neuro-psychopharmacology. Waikoloa, Hawaii, December 9–13, 2001.

[20] Davis LL, Kabel D, Patel D, et al. Valproate as an antidepressant in major depressive disorder. Psychopharmacol Bull 2004;32(4):647–52.

[21] Petty F, Davis LL, Nugent AL, et al. Valproate therapy for chronic, combat-induced posttraumatic stress disorder. J Clin Psychopharmacol 2002;22(1):100–1.

[22] Gyulai L, Bowden CL, McElroy SL, et al. Maintenance efficacy of divalproex in the prevention of bipolar depression. Neuropsychopharmacology 2003;28(7):1374–82.

[23] Bowden CL, Calabrese JR, McElroy SL, et al. A randomized, placebo-controlled 12-month trial of divalproex and lithium in treatment of outpatients with bipolar I disorder. Arch Gen Psychiatry 2000;57:481–9.

[24] Bowden CL, Janicak PG, Orsulak P, et al. Relationship of serum valproate concentration to response in mania. Am J of Psychiatry 1996;153(6):765–70.

[25] Luchins DJ, Klass D, Hanrahan P, et al. Computerized monitoring of valproate and physician responsiveness to laboratory studies as a quality indicator. Psychiatr Serv 2000; 51(9):1179–81.

[26] DeVane CL. Pharmacokinetics, drug interactions, and tolerability of valproate. Psycho-pharmacol Bull 2003;37(S2):25–42.

[27] Acharya S, Bussel JB. Hematologic toxicity of sodium valproate. J Pediatr Hematol Oncol 2000;22(1):62–5.

[28] Ketter TA, Wang PW, Post RM. Carbamazepine and oxcarbazepine. In: Schatzberg A, Nemeroff C, editors. Textbook of psychopharmacology. Washington (DC): American Psychiatric Publishing; 1998. p. 581–606.

[29] Keck PE Jr, Mendlwicz J, Calabrese JR, et al. A review of randomized, controlled clinical trials in acute mania. J Affect Disord 2000;59(S1):S31–7.

[30] Weisler RH, Kalali AH, Ketter TA, SPD 417 Study Group. A multicenter, randomized, double-blind, placebo-controlled trial of extended release carbamazepine capsules as monotherapy for bipolar disorder patients with manic or mixed episodes. J Clin Psychiat 2004;65(4):478–84.

[31] Ballenger JC, Post RM. Carbamazepine in manic-depressive illness: a new treatment. Am J Psychiatry 1980;137(7):782–90.

[32] Ernst CL, Goldberg JF. Antidepressant properties of anticonvulsant drugs for bipolar disorder. J Clin Psychopharmacol 2003;23(2):182–92.

[33] Post RM, Uhde TW, Roy-Byrne PP, et al. Antidepressant effects of carbamazepine. Am J Psychiatry 1986;143(1):29–34.

[34] Post RM, Denicoff KD, Frye MA, et al. Re-evaluating carbamazepine prophylaxis in bipolar disorder. Br J Psychiatry 1997;170:202–4.

[35] Okuma T, Inanage K, Otsuki S, et al. A preliminary double-blind study on the efficacy of carbamazepine in prophylaxis of manic-depressive illness. Psychopharmacology (Berl) 1981; 73:95–6.

[36] Greil W, Kleindienst N, Erazo N, et al. Differential response to lithium and carbamazepine in the prophylaxis of bipolar disorder. J Clin Psychopharmacol 1998;18(6):455–60.

[37] Bowden CL. Acute and maintenance treatment with mood stabilizers. Int J Neuro-psychopharmacol 2003;6:269–75.

[38] Denicoff KD, Smith-Jackson EE, Disney ER, et al. Comparative prophylactic efficacy of lithium, carbamazepine, and the combination in bipolar disorder. J Clin Psychiatry 1997; 58(11):470–8.

[39] Hellewell JS. Oxcarbazepine (Trileptal) in the treatment of bipolar disorders: review of efficacy and tolerability. J Affect Disord 2002;72(S1):S23–34.

[40] Emrich HM. Studies with oxcarbazepine in acute mania. Int Clin Psychopharmacol 1990;(S5):83–8.

[41] Trileptal [package insert]. East Hanover, NJ: Novartis Pharmaceuticals Corp; 2000.

[42] Muzina DJ, El-Sayegh S, Calabrese JR. Antiepileptic drugs in psychiatry-focus on randomized controlled trial. Epilepsy Res 2002;50(1–2):195–202.

[43] Physicians' Desk Reference. 59th edition. Montvale (NJ): Thomson PDR; 2005.

[44] Van Parys JA, Meinardi H. Survey of 260 epileptic patients treated with oxcarbazepine (Trileptal) on a named-patient basis. Epilepsy Res 1994;19(1):79–85.

[45] Bowden C, Calabrese R, Ascher J, et al. Spectrum of efficacy of lamotrigine in bipolar disorder: overview of double-blind, placebo-controlled studies. Abstracts of the 2000 Annual Meeting of the American College of Neuropsychopharmacology (ACNP). Nashville, TN: ACNP.

[46] Bowden CL. Lamotrigine in the treatment of bipolar disorder. Expert Opin Pharmacother 2002;10:1513–9.

[47] Calabrese JR, Bowden CL, Sachs GS, et al. A double-blind placebo-controlled study of lamotrigine monotherapy in outpatients with bipolar I depression. J Clin Psychiatry 1999;60: 79–88.

[48] Frye MA, Ketter TA, Kimbrell TA, et al. A placebo-controlled study of lamotrigine and gabapentin monotherapy in refractory mood disorders. J Clin Psychopharmacol 2000;20: 607–14.

[49] Bowden CL, Calabrese JR, Sachs G, et al. A placebo-controlled 18-month trial of lamotrigine and lithium maintenance treatment in recently manic or hypomanic patients with bipolar I disorder. Arch Gen Psychiatry 2003;60:392–400.

[50] Calabrese JR, Bowden CL, Sachs G, et al. A placebo-controlled 18-month trial of lamotrigine and lithium maintenance treatment in recently depressed patients with bipolar i disorder. J Clin Psychiatry 2003;64:1013–24.

[51] Calabrese JR, Vieta E, Shelton MD. Latest maintenance data on lamotrigine in bipolar disorder. Eur Neuropsychopharmacol 2003;13:S57–66.

[52] Calabrese JR, Suppes T, Bowden CL, et al. A double-blind placebo-controlled prophylaxis study of lamotrigine in rapid cycling bipolar disorder. J Clin Psychiatry 2000;61:841–50.

[53] Lamictal [package insert]. Research Triangle Park. NC: GlaxoSmithKline; 2003.

[54] Cunnington MC. The International Lamotrigine Pregnancy Registry Update for the Epilepsy Foundation. Epilepsia 2004;45(11):1468.

[55] Gidal B, Garnett W, Graves N. Epilepsy. In: Dipiro J, Talbert RL, Yee G, et al, editors. Pharmacotherapy—a pathophysiologic approach. New York, NY: McGraw-Hill; 2002. p. 1031–6.

[56] McElroy S, Keck PE Jr. Topiramate. In: Schatzberg A, Nemeroff C, editors. Textbook of chopharmacology. Washington (DC): American Psychiatric Publishing; 1998. p. 627–36.

[57] McIntyre RS, Mancini DA, McCann S, et al. Topiramate versus bupropion SR when added to mood stabilizer therapy for the depressive phase of bipolar disorder: a preliminary single-blind study. Bipolar Disord 2002;4(3):207–13.

[58] Vieta E, Goikolea JM, Olivares JM, et al. 1-year follow-up of patients treated with risperidone and topiramate for a manic episode. J Clin Psychiatry 2003;64(7):834–9.

[59] Frye M. Gabapentin. In: Schatzberg A, Nemeroff C, editors. Textbook of psychopharmacology. Washington (DC): American Psychiatric Publishing; 1998. p. 607–13.

[60] Pande AC, Crockatt JG, Janney CA, et al. Gabapentin in bipolar disorder: a placebo-controlled trial of adjunctive therapy. Gabapentin Bipolar Disorder Study Group. Bipolar Disord 2000;2(3 Pt 2):249–55.

[61] Pande AC, Davidson JR, Jefferson JW, et al. Treatment of social phobia with gabapentin: a placebo-controlled study. J Clin Psychopharmacol 1999;19(4):341–8.

[62] Kanba S, Yagi G, Kamijima K, et al. The first open study of zonisamide, a novel anticonvulsant, shows efficacy in mania. Prog Neuropsychopharmacol 1994;18(4):707–15.

[63] Gadde KM, Franciscy DM, Wagner HR II, et al. Zonisamide for weight loss in obese adults: a randomized controlled trial. JAMA 2003;289(14):1820–5.

[64] Kaufman K. Monotherapy treatment of bipolar disorder with levetiracetam. Epilepsy Behav 2004;5(6):1017–20.

[65] Grunze H, Langosch J, Born C, et al. Levetiracetam in the treatment of acute mania: an open add-on study with an on-off-on design. J Clin Psychiatry 2003;64(7):781–4.

[66] Fischer JH, Patel TV, Fischer PA. Fosphenytoin: clinical pharmacokinetics and comparative advantages in the acute treatment of seizures. Clin Pharmacokinet 2003; 42(1):33–58.

[67] Kalinowsky LB, Putnam TJ. Attempts at treatment of schizophrenia and other non-epileptic psychoses with Dilantin. Arch Neurol Psychiatry 1943;49:414–20.

[68] Mishory A, Yaroslavsky Y, Bersudsky Y, et al. Phenytoin as an antimanic anticonvulsant: a controlled study. Am J Psychiatry 2000;157(3):463–5.

[69] Applebaum J, Levine J, Belmaker RH. Intravenous fosphenytoin in acute mania. J Clin Psychiatry 2003;64(4):408–9.

ELSEVIER
SAUNDERS

Psychiatr Clin N Am
28 (2005) 325–347

PSYCHIATRIC
CLINICS
OF NORTH AMERICA

Atypical Antipsychotics for Bipolar Disorder

Lakshmi N. Yatham, MBBS, FRCPC

Mood Disorders Clinical Research Unit, University of British Columbia,
Room 2C7-2255 Wesbrook Mall, Vancouver, BC V6T 2A1, Canada

The term atypical antipsychotic is used to describe a group of medications that have efficacy in treating psychosis but have little or no propensity to cause extrapyramidal symptoms (EPS) [1]. Atypical antipsychotic agents have higher affinity to 5-HT2A receptors than to dopamine D2 receptors, and it has been argued that this unique property gives these medications a lower propensity toward EPS and increased efficacy against negative symptoms [2,3]. Clozapine is the prototype of atypical antipsychotic agents. Although clozapine was used initially to treat psychosis as early as the 1970s, its use was rapidly abandoned because of deaths associated with agranulocytosis [4]. The demonstration of the benefit of clozapine in treating refractory psychosis in the 1980s [5] fuelled development of other atypical antipsychotic agents.

During the past decade, several atypical antipsychotic agents, including risperidone, olanzapine, quetiapine, ziprasidone, aripiprazole, and amisulpiride, became available in various parts of the world. Case reports and open studies documenting the usefulness of atypical antipsychotic agents in bipolar disorder provided a much-needed impetus for the pharmaceutical industry to embark on comprehensive clinical trial development programs to examine the efficacy of atypical antipsychotic agents in various phases of bipolar disorder [6,7]. Olanzapine was the first to be examined in double-blind, placebo-controlled trials for treatment of acute mania [8,9] and bipolar depression [10] and for prevention of mood episodes [11]. Trials of risperidone [12–14], quetiapine [15,16], ziprasidone [17,18], and aripiprazole [19,20] examined the antimanic efficacy of the other atypical antipsychotic agents. To date only quetiapine has been examined for its antidepressant properties [21] and aripiprazole for prophylaxis [22] in double-blind,

E-mail address: yatham@interchange.ubc.ca

placebo-controlled studies. No double-blind trials to date have reported on the efficacy of clozapine or amisulpiride in bipolar disorder.

The results of double-blind trials suggest that the atypical antipsychotic agents examined to date have antimanic, antidepressant, and prophylactic properties in bipolar disorder. Atypical antipsychotic agents reduce dopamine transmission through blockade of or partial agonism for dopamine D2 receptors; this action might explain their antimanic effect, because mania is reported to be associated with dopaminergic hyperactivity [23]. More importantly, the ability of atypical antipsychotic agents to block or down-regulate 5-HT2A receptors [24] may explain their antidepressant effect. Recent positron emission tomography studies have shown that down-regulation of 5-HT2A receptors may be associated with relief or prevention of depressive symptoms [25,26].

This article reviews the data from double-blind, controlled trials investigating the efficacy of atypical antipsychotic agents in acute mania, in acute bipolar depression, and in continuation and maintenance treatment of bipolar disorder.

Acute mania

Placebo-controlled monotherapy studies

Each of the five atypical antipsychotic agents currently available in North America (ie, risperidone, olanzapine, quetiapine, ziprasidone, and aripiprazole) has been examined in at least two placebo-controlled, double-blind trials for treatment of acute mania [8,9,12–20]. All studies with the exception of ziprasidone studies [17,18] used changes in the Young Mania Rating Scale (YMRS) scores from the baseline to the endpoint as the primary measure of efficacy. The ziprasidone studies used the changes in Mania Rating Scale scores of the Schedule for Affective Disorders and Schizophrenia (MRS-SADS). All studies were of 3 weeks' duration except one study with olanzapine, which was 4 weeks, and the quetiapine studies, which continued for 12 weeks; the primary endpoint for these studies was the score at the end of week 3 using the last observation carried forward method. The entry criteria included a mania severity score of 20 or higher on the YMRS ($\geq$14 on the MRS for ziprasidone studies), and all studies excluded patients with substance abuse. Manic patients with and without psychotic features were included in all studies; patients with mixed episodes and rapid cycling were included in some studies but not in others. The design and results of these studies are summarized in Table 1.

Because of the similarity of these trials, comparative data from these trials are reviewed using the following clinically meaningful efficacy measures: (1) changes in the primary efficacy measure, (2) onset of action, (3) response rates, (4) remission rates, (5) patient subgroups, and (6) induction of depression.

Table 1
Studies of atypical antipsychotic agents as acute monotherapy versus placebo

Author Study duration, baseline YMRS/ MADRS or HAM-D	Treatments: daily dose in mg (mean)	n-value completed/ enrolled (%)	Onset of action	Reduction in YMRS total change versus baseline	% Responders (≥50% reduction in YMRS)	Reduction in HAM-D or MADRS change versus baseline	Most common side effects
Hirschfeld et al 2004 [12] 3 weeks YMRS total = 29; MADRS 9.5	RIS 1–6 (4.1) PBO	75/134 (56) 52/125	4 days	−11 −.0 $P < 0.001$	43 24 $P < 0.01$	−1.6 −0.1	EPS: RIS = PBO More somnolence, hyperkinesia, dyspepsia, nausea Weight gain: RIS > PBO + 1.6 versus −0.25 kg, $P < 0.001$
Khanna et al 2003 [13] 3 weeks YMRS total = 37; MADRS 5.4	RIS 1–6 (5.6) PBO	130/146 (89) 102/144 (71)	7 days	−22.4 −10 $P < 0.001$	73 36 $P < 0.001$	−3.2 −2.5 $P < 0.001$	EPS: RIS 35% versus PBO 6% Weight gain: RIS = PBO + 0.07 kg in both groups
Smulevich et al 2004 [14] 3 weeks YMRS total = 31.6	RIS 1–6 (4.2) PBO	137/154 (88.9) 119/140 (85)	7 days	−15.1 −9.4 $P < 0.001$	48 33 $P < 0.01$	−3.4 −2.3 $P < 0.001$	Mean ESRS, weight gain, and discontinuations because of AEs: RIS = PBO
Tohen et al 1999 [8] 3 weeks YMRS total = 28; HAM-2 = 13.3	OLZ 5–20 (14.9) PBO	43/70 (61.4) 24/69 (34.8) $P = 0.002$	21 days	−10.26 −4.88 $P = 0.02$	48.6 24.2 $P = 0.004$	−3.0 −2.9 $P = 0.87$	EPS: OLZ = PBO Significantly more somnolence, dry mouth, dizziness Weight gain: OLZ > PBO + 1.65 versus −0.44 kg, $P < 0.001$

(continued on next page)

Table 1 (continued)

Author Study duration, baseline YMRS/ MADRS or HAM-D	Treatments: daily dose in mg (mean)	n-value completed/ enrolled (%)	Onset of action	Reduction in YMRS total change versus baseline	% Responders (≥50% reduction in YMRS)	Reduction in HAM-D or MADRS change versus baseline	Most common side effects
Tohen et al 2000 [9] 4 weeks YMRS total = 29; HAM-D = 16.7	OLZ 5–20 (16.4) PBO	34/55 (61.8) 25/60 (41.7) P = 0.04	7 days	−14.78 −8.13 P < 0.001	64.8 42.9 P = 0.02	−7.83 −4.45 P = 0.09	EPS: OLZ = PBO Significantly more somnolence, dry mouth Weight gain: OLZ > PBO + 2.11 versus 0.45 kg, P = 0.002
McIntyre et al 2004 [16] 3-week data (12-week study) YMRS total = 33	QUE up to 800 mg/day (564) PBO	66/102 (64.7%) 61/101 (60.4%)	21 days	−12.29 −8.32 P = 0.009	42.6 35	−2.82 0.93 P < 0.005	Weight gain: QUE > PBO
Bowden et al 2004 [15] 3-week data (12-week study), YMRS total = 33	QUE up to 800 mg/day (649) PBO	97/107 (90.7%) 67/97 (69.1%)	21 days	−14.62 −6.71 P < 0.001	53.3 27.4	−1.55 −0.05	Weight gain, dry mouth, somnolence, and dizziness: QUE > PBO
Keck et al 2003 [17] 3 weeks SAD-C MRS = 27	ZIP 80–160 PBO	65/140 (46.4) 39/70 (55.7)	2 days	−12.4 −7.8 P < 0.005	50 35 P < 0.05	NR	EPS: ZIP = PBO More somnolence, headache, dizziness, hypertonia, nausea, akathisia Weight gain: No significant changes

Study	Medication	n/total (%)	Onset	Scale change	%		Adverse effects
Segal et al 2003 [18] 3 weeks SAD-C MRS = 26.3 MADRS = 12.7	ZIP 80–160 PBO	85/139 (61.1) 30/66 (45.4)	2 days	−11.12 −5.62 $P = 0.001$	46 29 $P < 0.05$	−3.74 −2.05	More somnolence, headache, dizziness, EPS, akathisia, nausea, tremor, abnormal vision, asthenia, constipation, dry mouth, and dystonia. Weight gain: No significant changes
Keck et al 2003 [19] 3 weeks YMRS total = 28.9	ARI 30 PBO	54/130 28/132	4 days	−8.2 −3.4 $P = 0.002$	40 19 $P < 0.01$	NR	ARI = PBO discontinuation rate and weight gain but EPS, nausea, and dyspepsia more common in ARI group
Hadjakis 2004 [20] 3 weeks YMRS total = 28.63	ARI 15–30 (27.6) PBO	75/137 (55) 71/135 (52)	4 days	−12.5 −7.2 $P < 0.001$	53 32 $P < 0.01$	−4.33 −3.2 $P = 0.18$	ARI = PBO in weight gain and discontinuation because of adverse events

Abbreviations: ARI, aripiprazole; EPS, extrapyramidal symptoms; ESRS, Extrapyramidal Symptom Rating Scale; HAM-D, Hamilton Depression Rating Scale; MADRS, Montgomery-Asberg Depression Rating Scale; NR, not reported; OLZ, olanzapine; *P*, p-value versus placebo; PBO, placebo; RIS, risperidone; YMRS, Young Mania Rating Scale; ZIP, ziprasidone.

Adapted from Yatham LN. Acute and maintenance treatment of bipolar mania: the role of atypical antipsychotics. Bipolar Disord 2003;5(Suppl 2):7–19.

Changes in the primary efficacy measure

Each of the 10 studies showed that the atypical antipsychotic agent was superior to placebo in treating acute manic symptoms as indicated by significantly greater reductions on the primary efficacy measure. In addition, a study that examined the efficacy of risperidone versus placebo versus haloperidol with a 3-week primary endpoint also showed superiority of risperidone in comparison with placebo [14]. The mean difference of reduction on primary efficacy measure between an atypical antipsychotic agent and placebo in these studies ranged from −3.97 to −12.4. The averages of the mean differences in the primary efficacy measure in the two studies for each of the atypical antipsychotic agents (or three studies for risperidone) were remarkably similar (−6.05 for olanzapine, −5.94 for quetiapine, −5.07 for aripiprazole, and −5.05 for ziprasidone), but risperidone had slightly larger reductions (−7.9). The greater average reduction for risperidone resulted mainly from a larger reduction in YMRS scores (−12.4) observed in the India study [13], which enrolled more severely ill manic patients than the other acute mania studies.

Onset of action

Medications that work faster may lead to savings in significant health care costs by reducing hospitalization days. The earliest day at which a medication separates from a placebo might indicate how quickly a medication works in treating manic symptoms. The earlier studies that examined the efficacy of atypical antipsychotic agents used day 7 as the first postrandomization measurement day, but more recent studies have used day 2. The first olanzapine study did not show separation from placebo until week 3 [8]. The starting dosage of olanzapine in this study was only 10 mg, however, which is somewhat lower than the dose clinicians routinely use for treating acute mania. In the second olanzapine study, which used 15 mg as the starting dose, separation from placebo was shown on day 7, the first postrandomization measurement date [9]. Risperidone studies used day 3 as the first measurement date. One study showed separation on that day [12]; the other showed separation on day 7 [13]. The quetiapine studies had very slow dose titration schedules (100 mg on day 1 increased by 100 mg/day until day 4 and to 600 mg on day 5). This slow titration schedule may, to some extent, have accounted for the lack of separation from placebo until day 21 in the quetiapine studies [15,16]. The combined analysis of two quetiapine monotherapy studies, however, revealed a separation from placebo on day 4 [27]. Both ziprasidone studies showed separation from placebo in changes in MRS scores on day 2 [17,18], and aripiprazole studies showed separation on day 4 [19,20].

Response rates

Clinicians are more interested in the number of patients who respond to a given agent than in the mean reductions in YMRS scores for a group of patients. Therefore all clinical trials report response rates, and the response is typically defined as a 50% or greater reduction on the primary efficacy measure score (YMRS or MRS) or "much or very much improvement" on the Clinical Global Impression–Improvement (CGI-I) Scale. The differences in response rates between an active agent and a placebo (placebo-corrected response rate) from each study for each agent should provide an estimate of true response to the medication.

The placebo-corrected response rates on YMRS ranged from 8% to 37%. The placebo-corrected response rates were similar in the monotherapy studies for olanzapine (24.4% and 21.9%) [8,9], ziprasidone (15% and 16.8%) [17,18], and aripiprazole (21% in both studies) [19,20], but the differences in response rates were substantial between the three studies for risperidone (15%, 19%, and 37%) [12–14] and for quetiapine (26% and 8%) [15,16]. The differences in the severity of mania in patients enrolled in the three risperidone studies may account for the differences in response rates, but the severity of mania was similar in the two quetiapine studies.

The mean placebo-corrected response rates (ie, the average response rates from placebo-controlled trials for each agent) were in the range of 16% to 23.3% (23.3% for risperidone, 23.2% for olanzapine, 17% for quetiapine, 21% for aripiprazole, and 15.9% for ziprasidone). Overall, the results of these studies suggest that there is an incremental response rate of about 20% to 25% with active medication over placebo.

Remission rates

Patients who meet criteria for response may still have significant manic symptoms, because response requires only a 50% reduction in rating scale scores. Remission should be the goal of therapy, but there is no consensus as to what constitutes remission. Furthermore, only the risperidone, olanzapine, and quetiapine studies reported remission rates; the aripiprazole and ziprasidone studies did not.

Remission rates will probably vary depending on the definition used. Olanzapine and quetiapine monotherapy studies used a score of 12 or lower on YMRS to define remission. Using this definition, remission rates were 20% to 25% higher with olanzapine than with placebo at weeks 3 [8] and 4 [9], respectively. In the two studies comparing quetiapine with placebo, the remission rates for quetiapine were 4% and 24.5%, respectively, higher than placebo at week 3 and 23.4% and 35.5%, respectively, higher than placebo at week 12 [15,16]. The two risperidone studies using a more stringent definition of 8 or lower on the YMRS and 12 or lower on the Montgomery-Asberg Depression Rating Scale (MADRS) reported remission rates that were 11% to 36%, respectively, higher than placebo at week 3 [12,13].

In a re-analysis of two olanzapine monotherapy trials, remission was defined as both a YMRS and Hamilton Depression Rating Scale-21 Item (HAM-D$_{21}$) score of 7 or lower, plus a Clinical Global Impression Scale-Bipolar version score of 2 or lower. Using this more stringent definition, remission rates with olanzapine were noted to be significantly greater (9%) than with placebo [28].

Patient subgroups

The proportion of patients with mixed episodes varied, and only a few studies reported on the outcome for mixed patients separately. Both the placebo-controlled trials of olanzapine monotherapy included patients with mixed episodes, and both studies showed that the magnitude of change in YMRS scores in patients with mixed episodes was similar to that in patients with manic episodes [8,9]. Both the quetiapine studies [15,16] and two of the risperidone studies [12,14] excluded mixed patients. The third risperidone study, which included mixed patients, reported similar reductions in YMRS scores in patients with mixed and manic episodes (-28.7 versus -22.5); however, only 6% of patients in this study had a mixed episode [13]. In the trial with ziprasidone, patients in the manic and mixed subgroups had comparable improvements in MRS scale scores (-13.1 and -11.2) [17]. The aripiprazole studies included a significant number of mixed-episode patients, but the results for these patients were not reported separately [19,20].

Most studies with risperidone and both quetiapine studies excluded patients with rapid cycling. The aripiprazole study included patients with rapid cycling, but results were not reported. Although both olanzapine studies included this patient subgroup, only one study reported specific results. Changes in YMRS scores were significantly greater with olanzapine in 45 patients with a rapid cycling course than with placebo (-13.9 versus -4.1; $P = 0.01$) [8].

All the studies included patients with and without psychotic features. In general, the results suggested that the magnitude of improvement in YMRS scores was similar in patients with and without psychotic features [8,9,12,13,15,16] and were significantly greater than the improvement seen with placebo.

Induction of depressive symptoms

Although conventional antipsychotic agents have been reported to induce depressive symptoms in manic patients [29], there is no evidence to suggest that atypical antipsychotic agents have the same liability. In one of the olanzapine studies that reported this outcome, the proportion of patients in the olanzapine group who experienced a clinically detectable worsening of depression was similar to that in the placebo group (11.1% versus 17.9%; $P = 0.42$) [9]. Similarly, mean reductions in MADRS scores in the risperidone group were greater in one study [13] and similar to the placebo group in the other study [12], suggesting that risperidone also does not have a propensity to induce depression. Both quetiapine studies found greater mean reductions in MADRS scores in the quetiapine group than in the placebo group and that the incidence of treatment-emergent depression was similar in the quetiapine and the placebo groups [15,16]. The aripiprazole and ziprasidone studies have not reported on this outcome measure.

Double-blind active comparator studies for acute mania

Studies that compared atypical antipsychotic monotherapy with conventional antipsychotic or lithium or divalproex monotherapy are summarized in Table 2 [14–16,30–35].

With the exception of ziprasidone, all atypical antipsychotic agents currently available in North America have been compared with haloperidol monotherapy for treatment of acute mania. The olanzapine and aripiprazole studies had no placebo groups; the risperidone and quetiapine studies included placebo comparator groups. The primary endpoint for acute mania was at 6 weeks in the olanzapine study [34] and at 3 weeks in the risperidone [14], quetiapine [16], and aripiprazole [35] studies. None of the studies showed any significant differences in changes on the YMRS scores or in response rates between the atypical antipsychotic agent and haloperidol. In general, the incidence of EPS was higher in the haloperidol group in all studies.

Olanzapine [31], risperidone [30], and quetiapine [15] were also compared with lithium monotherapy. The results showed that each of these atypical antipsychotic agents is as effective as lithium monotherapy in treating acute mania. Olanzapine was compared with divalproex in two double-blind studies with conflicting results [32,33]. In one trial of 248 patients, changes in YMRS total scores were significantly greater with olanzapine (-13.4) than with divalproex (-10.4, $P < 0.03$) [32]. In a smaller trial (n = 120), there was no significant difference between the two treatments [33].

The placebo-controlled trials of atypical antipsychotic agents show similar mean changes in YMRS scores and response rates, suggesting that there are no significant differences in the efficacy of the various atypical antipsychotic agents for treating acute mania. The best way to establish similarity or difference in efficacy, however, is to conduct a head-to-head comparator study, and only one such study has been conducted to date for acute mania. In this 3-week trial, olanzapine was compared with risperidone in the treatment of 329 patients with nonpsychotic acute mania [36]. Results showed no differences in changes in YMRS scores or responder rates between the two groups. The mean improvement in MADRS score was significantly greater with olanzapine than with risperidone, but because the difference in score was only one point, the clinical significance of this finding remains unclear.

Combination therapy studies

The combination of an atypical antipsychotic agent and a mood stabilizer is commonly used in clinical practice, and studies suggest that up to 80% of patients receive combination therapy [37–39]. Because of the widespread use

Table 2
Studies of atypical antipsychotic agents as acute monotherapy versus mood stabilizers or conventional antipsychotics

Author study duration baseline YMRS/MADRS or HAM-D	Treatments: daily dose in mg (mean)	n-value completed/ enrolled (%)	Reduction in YMRS total change versus baseline	% Responders ($\geq 50\%$ reduction in YMRS)	Reduction in HAM-D or MADRS change versus baseline	Most common side effects
Segal et al 1998 [30] 4 weeks YMRS total = 27	RIS 6 HAL 10 Li 800–1200	13/15 (86.7) 12/15 (80) 14/15 (93.3)	−16.2 −18.2 −12.7 $P = 0.35$	NR	NR	EPS: RIS = HAL > Li, $P = 0.01$
Smulevich et al 2004 [14] 3 weeks YMRS total = 31.7 MADRS total = 6.7	RIS 1–6 (4.2) HAL 2–12 (8)	137/154 (88.9) 130/154 (84.4)	−15.1 −13.9 $P = $ NS	48 47	−4.0 −2.9 $P < 0.05$	More EPS in HAL group compared with RIS
Berk et al 1999 [31] 4 weeks MAS = 35	OLZ 10 Li 800	14/15 (93) 12/15 (80)	−24.9 −21.9 $P = 0.315$	NR	NR	EPS: OLZ = Li
Tohen et al 2002 [32] 3 weeks YMRS total = 28; HAM-D = 14.1	OLZ 5–20 (17.4) DVP 500–2500 (1401.2)	86/125 (68.8) 81/126 (64.3) $P = $ ns	−13.4 −10.4 $P < 0.03$	54.4 42.3 $P < 0.058$	−4.9 −3.5 $P = 0.31$	EPS: OLZ = DVP OLZ: Significantly more dry mouth, increased appetite, somnolence; DVP: Significantly more nausea Weight gain: OLZ > DVP + 2.5 kg versus + 0.9 kg, $P < 0.001$

Study	Treatment				Comments
Zajecka et al 2002 [33] 3-week data (12-week study) YMR total = 32.3, DVP 30.8, P = 0.046; HAM-D = 15.0	OLZ 10-20 (14.7) DVP 20 mg/kg/d-20 mg/kg/d + 1000 (2115)	38/57 (67) 45/63 (71)	-16.6 -14.9 $P = 0.21^a$	NR	-8.1 -6.7 P = 0.22	EPS: OLZ = DVP OLZ: Significantly more somnolence, rhinitis, edema, speech disorder Weight gain: OLZ > DVP + 4.0 kg versus + 2.5 kg, P = 0.049
Tohen et al 2003[34] 6-week data (12-week study) YMRS total = 30.9 HAM-D = 8.04	OLZ 5-20 HAL 3-15	166/234 (70.9) 141/219 (64.4)	-21.3 -23.5	52.1 46.1 (remission rates P = 0.15)	-2.8 -1.8	Somnolence, dizziness and weight gain: OLZ > HAL. EPS and increased salivation: HAL > OLZ
McIntyre et al 2004 [16] 3-week data (12-week study) YMRS total = 33	QUE up to 800 (564) HAL 2-8	66/102 (64.7) 77/99 (77.8)	-12.29 -15.71	42.6 56.1	-2.82 -2.28	EPS: HAL > QUE
Bowden et al 2004 [15] 3-week data (12-week study) YMRS total = 33	QUE up to 800 (649) Li	97/107 (90.7) 84/98 (85.7)	-14.62 -15.2	53.3 53.1	-1.55 -1.26	Tremor: Li > QUE
Bourin et al. 2003 [35] 3-week data (12-week study) YMRS total = 31.23	ARI 15-30 (22.6) HAL 10-15 (11.7)	134/175 (76.6) 95/172 (55.2)	-15.7 -15.67	50.9 42.6	-3.12 -1.57	EPS: ARI < HAL

Abbreviations: ARI, aripiprazole; DVP, divalproex; EPS, extrapyramidal symptoms; HAL, haloperidol; HAM-D, Hamilton Depression Rating Scale; Li, lithium; MADRS, Montgomery-Asberg Depression Rating Scale; MAS, mania scale; MS, mood stabilizers; NR, not reported; OLZ, olanzapine; P, p-value versus comparator; PBO, placebo; QUE, quetiapine; RIS, risperidone; YMRS, Young Mania Rating Scale; ZIP, ziprasidone.

^{a} Corrected for baseline differences.

Adapted from Yatham LN. Acute and maintenance treatment of bipolar mania: the role of atypical antipsychotics. Bipolar Disord 2003;5(Suppl 2):7-19.

of combination therapy, a number of recent studies compared the efficacy of an atypical antipsychotic agent (olanzapine in one study, risperidone in two studies, and quetiapine in three studies) plus a mood stabilizer with a mood stabilizer plus placebo for treating acute mania [40–45]. The duration of these studies varied from 3 to 6 weeks. The results of these studies are summarized in Table 3.

All six studies showed numerically greater reductions in the primary efficacy measure of YMRS or MRS scores, but only four studies [40,41,43,45] showed statistical superiority of combination therapy over mood stabilizer monotherapy. In the failed risperidone study, when patients treated with carbamazepine (which reduced the plasma concentration of risperidone by 40%) were excluded, YMRS total scores at endpoint were significantly greater with risperidone than with placebo (mean difference, -5.4; $P = 0.047$). This result suggests that carbamazepine induction of risperidone metabolism may have accounted for the failure of this study on the primary efficacy measure [42]. In the failed quetiapine study, the combination group had numerically greater reductions in YMRS scores, but the differences were not significant because of the excellent response to a mood stabilizer alone in this study population. The combined analysis of the two quetiapine studies showed that changes in YMRS scores were significantly greater in the combination-therapy group than in the mood stabilizer plus placebo group [44]. Overall, given that there are two positive studies with quetiapine, and that the combined analysis of two large studies also showed positive result, it is likely that adding quetiapine to a mood stabilizer does provide additional benefit in treating acute manic symptoms. Mood stabilizer–corrected response rates to risperidone (18%–23%), olanzapine (23%), and quetiapine (14.1%, 22%–34%) plus mood stabilizer were on average about 20% higher than with mood stabilizer plus placebo, indicating that the combination treatment provides a clinically meaningful increase in response rates.

In all studies, weight gain was more common with combination therapy than with mood stabilizer monotherapy. Somnolence and dry mouth were more common with olanzapine and quetiapine; EPSs were more common with risperidone in one study [13].

Acute bipolar depression

Although bipolar patients experience depressive symptoms three times more commonly than mania [46], only two studies examined the efficacy of atypical antipsychotic agents in the treatment of acute bipolar depression in double-blind, placebo-controlled trials [10,21].

Olanzapine

As with mania, olanzapine was the first atypical antipsychotic agent to be assessed for its efficacy in acute bipolar I depression [10]. Eight hundred thirty-three patients were randomly assigned to olanzapine, 5 to 20 mg/day (n = 370), placebo (n = 377), or olanzapine plus fluoxetine combination (OFC) (n = 86) for 8 weeks. Both olanzapine and OFC were significantly superior to placebo at all visits and at endpoint on the primary efficacy measure of reduction in depressive symptoms as measured by the MADRS. Further, OFC was superior to olanzapine from week 4 to week 8. Remission rates were 24.5% for the placebo group, 32.8% for the olanzapine group, and 48.8% for the OFC group. The incidence of manic switch was not different among the three groups (placebo 6.7%, olanzapine 5.7%, and OFC 6.7%). The adverse-event profile was similar for the olanzapine and OFC groups, with weight gain, somnolence, increased appetite, dry mouth, and asthenia occurring more commonly than in the placebo group. Nausea and diarrhea were more common in OFC group than in the olanzapine group.

Quetiapine

In contrast to the olanzapine study, patients in the quetiapine study included both bipolar I (66.9%) and bipolar II (33.1%) depressed patients who were randomly assigned to treatment with quetiapine, 300 mg/day (n = 172), quetiapine, 600 mg/day (n = 170), or placebo (n = 169) for 8 weeks [21]. Patients in the quetiapine group were started on 50 mg/day and titrated upwards so that the target dose was reached by day 4 in the 300-mg group and by day 8 in the 600-mg group. Both quetiapine groups separated from the placebo group on the primary efficacy measure of change in MADRS scores from week 1 to 8 including the endpoint. Response rates were significantly greater for quetiapine groups (56% for 600 mg and 55% for 300 mg) than in the placebo group (31%). The incidence of treatment-emergent mania was similar in the three groups (2.4%, 3.5%, and 4.1%, respectively). Treatment-emergent adverse events, such as dry mouth, sedation, somnolence, and dizziness, were more common in both quetiapine groups than in the placebo group, but no differences in EPS or sexual adverse events were observed among the groups.

Continuation and maintenance therapy

In contrast to the extensive evidence for the efficacy of atypical antipsychotic agents in treating acute mania, the evidence for their efficacy in the continuation and maintenance treatment of bipolar disorder is limited, with the exception of olanzapine. No consensus exists as to what constitutes continuation or maintenance therapy for bipolar disorder. For the purpose of this article, continuation therapy studies are defined as those of at least 3 months' duration, and maintenance therapy studies are defined as those longer than 3 months. Because of the limited number of studies and the differences in study designs, each study is discussed separately.

Table 3
Studies of atypical antipsychotic agents as adjunct to mood stabilizers versus mood stabilizer monotherapy for acute treatment

Author study duration baseline YMRS/ MADRS/HAM-D	Treatments added to MS[a] daily dose in mg (mean)	n-value completed/ enrolled (%)	Reduction in YMRS total change versus baseline	% Responders (≥50% reduction in YMRS)	Reduction in HAM-D or MADRS change versus baseline	Most common side effects
Sachs et al 2002 [41] 3 weeks YMRS total = 28	RIS 1–6 (3.8) HAL 4–12 (6.2) PBO	34/52 (65) 25/53 (47) 26/51 (51)	−14.3, $P = 0.009$ −13.4, $P < 0.03$ −8.2	53[b], $P = 0.002$ 50[b], $P = 0.003$ 30%	NR	EPS: RIS = PBO; HAL > PBO, $P < 0.05$. Weight gain: RIS > PBO + 2.41 kg versus + 0.5 kg, $P < 0.004$. HAL = PBO + 0.14 kg
Yatham et al 2003 [42] 3 weeks YMRS total = 29; HAM-D = 8.4	RIS 1–6 (4) PBO	48/75 (64) 36/76 (48)	−14.5 (−15.2)[c], $P = 0.089$ −10.3 (−9.8)[c] ($P = 0.047$)	58.8 41.1 $P < 0.05$	−4.1 −2.1	EPS: RIS > PBO, $P = 0.013$. Weight gain: RIS > PBO + 1.7 kg versus + 0.5 kg, $P = 0.012$
Tohen et al 2002 [40] 6 weeks YMRS total = 22; HAM-D = 14.0	OLZ 5–20 (10.4) PBO	150/229 (69.9) 82/115 (71.3)	−13.11 −9.10 $P = 0.003$	67.7 44.7 $P < 0.001$	−4.98 −0.89 $P < 0.001$	EPS: OLZ = PBO. Significantly more somnolence, dry mouth, increased appetite, tremor, slurred speech. Weight gain: OLZ > PBO + 3.1 kg versus + 0.23 kg, $P < 0.001$

Study	Drug dose	N (%)				Adverse effects
Sachs et al 2003 [43] 3 weeks YMRS total = 31.3	QUE 200–800	56/90 (61.5)	−13.76	54.3	−3.36	>10%, QUE > PBO somnolence, dry mouth, asthenia, postural hypotension
	(580) PBO	49/100 (49.0)	−9.93	32.6	−2.79	
			P = 0.021	P = 0.005	P = 0.65	
Yatham et al 2004 [44] 3 weeks (combined data from a 3-week and a 6-week study) YMRS total = 32 MADRS = 11.75	QUE 200–800	133/197 (67.5)	−15.29	55.7	−3.69	QUE > PBO somnolence, dry mouth, asthenia, postural hypotension
	(580) PBO	114/205 (55.6)	−12.19	41.6	−3.06	
			P < 0.05	P < 0.01		
Delbello et al 2002 [45] 6 weeks YMRS total = 33	QUE 50–450	8/15 (53.3)	−24.5	87	NR	QUE > PBO sedation (80% versus 33%, P = 0.03)
	(432) PBO	14/15 (93.0)	−14	53		
			P = 0.03	P = 0.05		

Abbreviations: ARI, aripiprazole; DVP, divalproex; EPS, extrapyramidal symptoms; ESRS, Extrapyramidal Symptom Rating Scale; HAL, haloperidol; HAM-D, Hamilton Depression Rating Scale; Li, lithium; MADRS, Montgomery-Asberg Depression Rating Scale; MAS, mania scale; MS, mood stabilizers; NR, not reported; OLZ, olanzapine; P, p-value versus comparator; PBO, placebo; QUE, quetiapine; RIS, risperidone; YMRS, Young Mania Rating Scale; ZIP, ziprasidone.

Adapted from Yatham LN. Acute and maintenance treatment of bipolar mania: the role of atypical antipsychotics. Bipolar Disord 2003;5(Suppl 2):7–19.

[a] Usually lithium or divalproex (about 17% of patients in Yatham et al received carbamazepine).
[b] Much or very much improved on CGI change scale.
[c] Excluding carbamazepine subgroup.

Placebo-controlled monotherapy studies

A 1-year study examined the efficacy of olanzapine [11], and a 6-month study assessed the efficacy of aripiprazole [22] after an acute manic episode in the continuation/maintenance treatment of bipolar disorder. Quetiapine was examined only for continuation treatment of mania [15,16]. No placebo-controlled, double-blind studies reported on the efficacy of risperidone, ziprasidone, or clozapine in continuation/maintenance treatment.

Olanzapine

Patients with acute mania (n = 731) were treated with open-label olanzapine, 5 to 20 mg daily [11]. Patients who responded during a 6- to 12-week period and met criteria for randomization (n = 361) entered the double-blind phase and were randomly assigned to treatment with either olanzapine (n = 225) or placebo (n = 136) for 52 weeks. Approximately one third of patients had a mixed index episode, one fifth had psychotic features during the index manic episode, and about half of the patients in each group had a history of rapid cycling.

A significantly greater number of patients in the olanzapine group completed the study (53 versus 13), and fewer patients in the olanzapine group discontinued the study for lack of efficacy (64 versus 78) compared with the placebo group. Time to relapse into a mood episode (based on hospitalization, symptomatic rating scale criteria, or *Diagnostic and Statistical Manual IV* syndromic criteria) was significantly longer in the olanzapine group than in the placebo group. Significantly fewer patients in the olanzapine group than in the placebo group (46.7% versus 80.1%) had a relapse into a mood episode. Relapse rates were significantly lower in the olanzapine group than in the placebo group for manic episodes (16.4% versus 41.2%) and for depressive episodes (34.7% versus 47.8%).

There was no significant difference in the incidence of treatment-emergent EPS symptoms or tardive dyskinesia between the two groups. A significantly greater proportion of patients in the olanzapine group reported weight gain, akathisia, and fatigue. Insomnia was more common in the placebo group. Patients in the olanzapine group gained 3 kg during the open-label phase and 1 kg during the double-blind phase; patients in the placebo group lost 2 kg.

Aripiprazole

Patients with acute mania or mixed episode were treated with open-label aripiprazole, 15 to 30 mg/day, for 6 to 18 weeks, and those who met criteria for stabilization (ie, a YMRS score of 10 or lower and a MADRS score of 13 or lower for four consecutive visits or 6 weeks) were randomly assigned to double-blind maintenance treatment with aripiprazole (n = 78) or placebo (n = 83) for 26 weeks [22]. Time to relapse of a mood episode, defined as a discontinuation from study because of lack of efficacy, was significantly longer for the aripiprazole group than for the placebo group. Fewer patients in the aripiprazole group (24%) than in the placebo group (43%) had a relapse of a mood episode ($P = 0.013$). A subanalysis showed that the difference between the two groups was significant for manic but not for depressive relapses. No significant differences were noted between the two groups in frequency of adverse events such as EPS, weight gain, or prolactin levels.

Quetiapine versus placebo versus haloperidol

Patients with acute mania were randomly assigned to quetiapine (n = 102), placebo (n = 101), or haloperidol (n = 99) for acute (3 weeks) and continuation (12 weeks) treatment [16]. The number of patients meeting criteria for remission on YMRS increased from week 3 to week 12. A significantly greater proportion of patients in the quetiapine (61.4%) and haloperidol (63.3%) groups remitted by week 12, when compared with the placebo group (38%). The quetiapine patients had significantly greater reductions on MADRS scores (−3.31) compared with the placebo group (−0.68), but no significant difference was observed between the haloperidol (−1.85) and the placebo groups. The mean daily quetiapine dose in responders during the last week was 531 mg/day, and the haloperidol dose was 4.9 mg/day. Somnolence was more common in the quetiapine group, and EPS were more common in the haloperidol group than in the placebo group.

Quetiapine versus placebo versus lithium

The efficacy of quetiapine (n = 107) was examined in the continuation treatment of mania (12 weeks) in comparison with placebo (n = 97) and lithium (n = 98) [15]. A significantly greater number of patients in the quetiapine (67.3%) and lithium (68.4%) groups completed the study compared with the placebo group (36.1%). Remission rates on YMRS at week 12 were similar in the quetiapine (69.2%) and lithium (72.4%) groups and were significantly greater than in the placebo group (33.7%). Reductions in MADRS scores were also similar in the quetiapine (−1.49) and lithium (−1.83) groups and were greater than in the placebo group (+1.21). The mean daily dose of quetiapine in responders during the last week of treatment was 651 mg/day. Dry mouth, somnolence, weight gain, and dizziness were more common in the quetiapine group. Tremor was more common in the lithium group.

Double-blind active comparator monotherapy studies

Olanzapine was examined in comparison to lithium [47] and to divalproex [48] in 1-year maintenance therapy studies. Olanzapine [34], risperidone [14], aripiprazole [35], and quetiapine [15,16] were examined in 3-month continuation therapy studies.

Olanzapine versus lithium

Patients with bipolar I disorder who had a history of at least two manic/ mixed episodes within the past 6 years and were currently in an acute manic or mixed episode were treated with a combination of open-label olanzapine and lithium for 6 to 12 weeks [47]. Those with a history of intolerance or inadequate response to lithium or olanzapine were excluded. Subjects meeting remission criteria during the open-label period entered the double-blind taper period of 4 weeks, during which either lithium or olanzapine was tapered and discontinued, and the subjects continued with double-blind monotherapy with either of those agents for the remaining 48 weeks. More than 90% of patients in both groups had an index manic episode, and only 3% of patients in each group had a history of rapid cycling.

Of the 543 patients treated in the open-label phase, 431 achieved remission and were randomly assigned to double-blind monotherapy with olanzapine (n = 217) or lithium (n = 214). A significantly greater number of olanzapine-treated patients than lithium-treated patients completed the trial (46.5% versus 32.7%). Similarly, time to discontinuation for any reason was significantly longer for the olanzapine group than for the lithium group. There was a trend for the olanzapine group to have lower rates of relapse into any mood episode based on symptomatic rating scale criteria than the lithium group (30% versus 38.8%; $P = 0.055$). There was no significant difference in depressive relapse rates (16.5% versus 15.5%; $P = 0.89$), but significantly fewer olanzapine-treated patients than lithium-treated patients had relapse into manic/mixed episodes (14% versus 28%; $P < 0.001$). The rates of discontinuation for adverse events were lower with olanzapine than with lithium (18.9% versus 25.7%), but the rates of lack of efficacy were similar (14.3% versus 15.9%).

There was no significant difference between the two groups in treatment-emergent EPS based on rating scales or patient reporting. Among patient-reported adverse events, depression and hypersomnia were more common in the olanzapine group, and insomnia, nausea, and worsening of mania were more common in the lithium group. Patients taking olanzapine gained 2.74 kg during the open-label phase and another 1.8 kg in the double-blind phase; those taking lithium lost 1.4 kg.

Olanzapine versus divalproex sodium

Patients with acute mania (n = 251) were randomly assigned to olanzapine, 5 to 20 mg/day, or divalproex, 500 to 2500 mg/day for a 3-week acute phase and a 44-week maintenance phase [48]. Overall, no significant differences in syndromic or symptomatic relapse into a mood episode, a manic episode, or a depressive episode were noted between the two groups. Although the median time to remission of mania was significantly shorter in the olanzapine group than in the divalproex group, the rates of remission into mania at 47 weeks using the last observation carried forward method were not significantly different between the two groups. Treatment-emergent events such as weight gain, somnolence, dry mouth, increased appetite, and akathisia were more common in the olanzapine group. The incidence of nausea and nervousness was higher in the divalproex group.

Olanzapine versus haloperidol

A 12-week study had two phases: a 6-week acute phase, and another 6-week maintenance-of-response phase [34]. Of the 453 patients who entered the 6-week acute phase, 298 met criteria and entered the maintenance-of-response phase for treatment with olanzapine (n = 160) or haloperidol (n = 138) [34]. No differences were observed in relapse rates into a mood episode, a manic episode, or a depressive episode based on symptomatic or syndromal criteria, nor were there differences in time to relapse between the two groups. Response rates based on YMRS scores were 96.3% for the olanzapine group and 94.1% for the haloperidol group ($P = 0.42$). EPS were significantly more common in the haloperidol group. Weight gain, somnolence, and dizziness were more common in the olanzapine group.

Risperidone versus haloperidol

A double-blind 12-week trial compared the efficacy of risperidone (n = 154) versus haloperidol (n = 144) for acute and continuation treatment of mania [14]. This study had a placebo comparator group (n = 140) for the first 3 weeks. Patients with acute mania were treated with 1 to 6 mg of risperidone or 2 to 12 mg of haloperidol.

Ninety patients in the risperidone group and 64 patients in the haloperidol group entered the continuation phase (ie, 4 to 12 weeks of double-blind treatment). Of these, 77 (86%) in the risperidone group and 56 (88%) in the haloperidol group completed the 12 weeks of treatment. There were no significant differences between the two groups for discontinuation caused by adverse events (6% in the risperidone group versus 5% in the haloperidol group) or lack of efficacy (2% versus 0%, respectively). The mean reductions in YMRS scores (-28.7 ± 7.9 versus -27.3 ± 7.3) and the proportion of patients that maintained response from week 3 (98% versus 100%) were similar in the risperidone and haloperidol groups. An additional 83% of patients in the risperidone group and 89% of patients in the haloperidol group who had not met criteria for response at week 3 achieved response by week 12. The mean reductions in MADRS scores were greater in the risperidone group at week 3 (-3.4 versus -2.8) but were similar to those in the haloperidol group at week 12 (-4.6 ± 4.8 versus -2.8 ± 6.1). Mean increases in Extrapyramidal Symptom Rating Scale (ESRS) scores were significantly greater at the 12-week endpoint in the haloperidol group than in the risperidone group. The mean weight gain was 1.4 ± 4.6 kg in the risperidone group and 0.8 ± 3.5 kg in the haloperidol group.

Aripiprazole versus haloperidol

The efficacy of aripiprazole was compared with haloperidol for acute (3 weeks) and continuation (4–12 weeks) treatment of mania [35]. Patients were randomly assigned to treatment with aripiprazole (n = 175) or haloperidol (n = 172) for a 3-week treatment. Of these, 87 patients (50.6%) in the haloperidol group and 129 patients (73.7%) in the aripiprazole group entered the continuation phase. About 90% of patients in both groups had an index manic episode, and rapid cyclers were excluded. Fifty patients (29.1%) in the haloperidol group and 89 patients (50.9%) in the aripiprazole group completed the study. Time to discontinuation for any reason and the proportion of patients who met criteria for response on YMRS were significantly greater for the aripiprazole group (49.7%) than for the haloperidol group (28.4%). As expected, the incidence of EPS was greater in the haloperidol group, but no differences were observed in weight change (+0.27 kg for aripiprazole and −0.1 kg for haloperidol) between the two groups.

Quetiapine versus haloperidol and quetiapine versus lithium

Because the studies comparing haloperidol, quetiapine, and lithium included a placebo comparator group [15,16], the details of these studies are described in the section on placebo-controlled continuation therapy studies.

Double-blind combination therapy studies

Olanzapine is the only atypical antipsychotic agent that has been examined in combination with a mood stabilizer in comparison to a mood stabilizer plus placebo in a double-blind trial [49]. Patients who met criteria for remission within 6 weeks of olanzapine plus lithium or valproate treatment for an acute manic episode were randomly assigned to receive double-blind olanzapine, 5–20 mg/day (n = 46), or placebo (n = 48) as add-on therapy to lithium/valproate for 18 months. Three times more patients in the combination group (31%) completed the trial compared with those in the mood stabilizer plus placebo group (10%) ($P = 0.014$). Time to discontinuation was longer in the combination group than in the monotherapy group (111 versus 82 days; $P = 0.049$), but the time to syndromic relapse into a mood episode, manic episode, or a depressive episode was not different between the two groups. Of the patients who were asymptomatic at entry into the relapse prevention phase, the time to symptomatic relapse into a mood episode was significantly longer for those receiving combination therapy than for those treated with monotherapy (median time to relapse: 163 versus 42 days, respectively; $P = 0.023$). There was no significant difference in the incidence of EPS in the two groups.

Summary

Atypical antipsychotic agents have been widely investigated for their efficacy in acute mania. The data to date suggest that olanzapine, risperidone, quetiapine, aripiprazole, and ziprasidone are effective, with no significant differences in antimanic efficacy among these agents. These agents are effective as an alternative to lithium or divalproex as monotherapy or in combination with these mood stabilizers. The data concerning their utility in acute bipolar depression and maintenance treatment of bipolar disorder are limited. The studies to date suggest that olanzapine has modest acute antidepressant properties but probably has efficacy comparable to lithium and divalproex in preventing manic and depressive episodes. Quetiapine seems to have robust antidepressant properties, but these data need to be replicated in further trials before quetiapine can be recommended as a first-line agent for acute bipolar depression. Aripiprazole has shown promise in preventing manic episodes in one 6-month study, but further studies with at least 1-year duration and larger sample sizes are needed before this agent can be recommended as a monotherapy for prophylaxis of bipolar disorder. It is currently unknown if risperidone, aripiprazole, and ziprasidone have any efficacy in treating acute bipolar depression. Similarly, long-term studies are needed to ascertain the role of risperidone, quetiapine, and ziprasidone in the maintenance treatment of bipolar disorder. Overall, the atypical antipsychotic agents as a group represent an effective and relatively safe addition to the armamentarium for the treatment of bipolar disorder.

References

[1] Jibson MD, Tandon R. New atypical antipsychotic medications. J Psychiatr Res 1998; 32(3–4):215–28.
[2] Kane JM. Newer antipsychotic drugs—a review of their pharmacology and therapeutic potential. Drugs 1993;46(4):585–93.
[3] Leysen D, Linders JTM, Ottenheijm HCJ. 5–HT2 antagonists: a concept for the treatment of schizophrenia. Curr Pharm Des 1997;3(4):367–90.
[4] Alvir JMJ, Lieberman JA, Safferman AZ, et al. Clozapine-induced agranulocytosis—incidence and risk factors in the United States. N Engl J Med 1993;329(3):162–7.
[5] Kane J, Honigfeld G, Singer J, et al. Clozapine for the treatment-resistant schizophrenic—a double-blind comparison with chlorpromazine. Arch Gen Psychiatry 1988;45(9): 789–96.
[6] Tohen M, Zarate CA Jr. Antipsychotic agents and bipolar disorder. J Clin Psychiatry 1998; 59(Suppl 1):38–48.
[7] Ghaemi SN, Sachs GS, Baldassano CF, et al. Acute treatment of bipolar disorder with adjunctive risperidone in outpatients. Can J Psychiatry 1997;42(2):196–9.
[8] Tohen M, Sanger TM, McElroy SL, et al. Olanzapine versus placebo in the treatment of acute mania. Olanzapine HGEH Study Group. Am J Psychiatry 1999;156(5):702–9.
[9] Tohen M, Jacobs TG, Grundy SL, et al. Efficacy of olanzapine in acute bipolar mania: a double-blind, placebo-controlled study. The Olanzipine HGGW Study Group. Arch Gen Psychiatry 2000;57(9):841–9.
[10] Tohen M, Vieta E, Calabrese J, et al. Efficacy of olanzapine and olanzapine-fluoxetine combination in the treatment of bipolar I depression. Arch Gen Psychiatry 2003;60(11): 1079–88.
[11] Tohen M, Bowden C, Calabrese J, et al. Olanzapine's efficacy for relapse prevention in bipolar disorder: a randomized double-blind placebo-controlled 12-month clinical trial. Bipolar Disord 2004;6:26–7.

[12] Hirschfeld RMA, Keck PE, Kramer M, et al. Rapid antimanic effect of risperidone monotherapy: a 3-week multicenter, double-blind, placebo-controlled trial. Am J Psychiatry 2004;161(6):1057–65.

[13] Khanna S, Vieta E, Lyons B, et al. Risperidone in the treatment of acute bipolar mania: a double-blind, placebo-controlled study of 290 patients. Eur Neuropsychopharmacol 2003; 13:S314–5.

[14] Smulevich A, Khanna S, Eerdekens M, et al., Acute and continuation risperidone monotherapy in bipolar mania: a 3 week placebo controlled trial followed by a 9-week double-blind trial of risperidone and haloperidol. Eur Neuropsychopharmacol, in press.

[15] Bowden CL, Grunze H, Mullen J, et al. A randomized double blind placebo controlled efficacy and safety study of quetiapine or lithium as monotherapy for mania in bipolar disorder. J Clin Psychiatry, in press.

[16] McIntyre R, Brecher M, Paulsson B. Quetiapine as monotherapy for bipolar mania: a double blind randomized parellel group placebo controlled trial. Eur Neuropsychopharmacol 2004, in press.

[17] Keck PE, Versiani M, Potkin S, et al. Ziprasidone in the treatment of acute bipolar mania: a three-week, placebo-controlled, double-blind, randomized trial. Am J Psychiatry 2003; 160(4):741–8.

[18] Segal S, Riesenberg RA, Ice K, et al. Ziprasidone in mania: a 21-day randomized, double-blind, placebo controlled trial. Eur Neuropsychopharmacol 2003;13:S345–6.

[19] Keck PE, Marcus R, Tourkodimitris S, et al. A placebo-controlled, double-blind study of the efficacy and safety of aripiprazole in patients with acute bipolar mania. Am J Psychiatry 2003;160(9):1651–8.

[20] Hadjakis WJ, Marcus R, Abou-Gharbia N, et al. Aripiprazole in acute mania: results from a second placebo-controlled study. Bipolar Disord 2004;6:39–40.

[21] Calabrese JR, Keck PE Jr, Macfadden W, et al. A randomized double blind placebo controlled trial of quetiapine in the treatment of bipolar I or II depression. Am J Psychiatry 2004, in press.

[22] Sanchez R, Marcus R, Carson WH, et al. Aripiprazole in the maintenance treatment of bipolar disorder. Eur Psychiatry 2004;19:204S.

[23] Yatham LN. Brain imaging investigations of dopaminergic pathways in mood disorders. In: Soares JC, editor. Brain imaging in affective disorders. New York: Marcel Dekker; 2003.

[24] Tarazi FI, Zhang KH, Baldessarini RJ. Long-term effects of olanzapine, risperidone, and quetiapine on serotonin 1A, 2A and 2C receptors in rat forebrain regions. Psychopharmacology (Berl) 2002;161(3):263–70.

[25] Yatham LN, Liddle PF, Dennie J, et al. Decrease in brain serotonin 2 receptor binding in patients with major depression following desipramine treatment: a positron emission tomography study with fluorine-18-labeled setoperone. Arch Gen Psychiatry 1999;56(8): 705–11.

[26] Yatham LN, Liddle PF, Shiah IS, et al. Effects of rapid tryptophan depletion on brain 5–HT2 receptors: a PET study. Br J Psychiatry 2001;178:448–53.

[27] Jones M, Huizar K. Randomised, double-blind, controlled data on the treatment of mania with quetiapine. Eur Psychiatry 2004;19:206S–7S.

[28] Chengappa KNR, Baker RW, Shao LX, et al. Rates of response, euthymia and remission in two placebo-controlled olanzapine trials for bipolar mania. Bipolar Disord 2003;5(1):1–5.

[29] Esparon J, Kolloori J, Naylor GJ, et al. Comparison of the prophylactic action of flupenthixol with placebo in lithium treated manic-depressive patients. Br J Psychiatry 1986; 148:723–5.

[30] Segal J, Berk M, Brook S. Risperidone compared with both lithium and haloperidol in mania: a double-blind randomized controlled trial. Clin Neuropharmacol 1998;21(3): 176–80.

[31] Berk M, Ichim L, Brook S. Olanzapine compared to lithium in mania: a double-blind randomized controlled trial. Int Clin Psychopharmacol 1999;14(6):339–43.

[32] Tohen M, Baker RW, Altshuler LL, et al. Olanzapine versus divalproex in the treatment of acute mania. Am J Psychiatry 2002;159(6):1011–7.

[33] Zajecka JM, Weisler R, Sachs G, et al. A comparison of the efficacy, safety, and tolerability of divalproex sodium and olanzapine in the treatment of bipolar disorder. J Clin Psychiatry 2002;63(12):1148–55.

[34] Tohen M, Goldberg JF, Arrillaga AMGP, et al. A 12-week, double-blind comparison of olanzapine vs haloperidol in the treatment of acute mania. Arch Gen Psychiatry 2003;60(12):1218–26.

[35] Bourin M, Auby P, Swanik S, et al. Aripiprazole vs. haloperidol for maintained treatment effect in acute mania. Eur Neuropsychopharmacol 2003;13:S333.

[36] Baker R, Zarate C Jr, Brown E, et al. A three-week comparison of olanzapine versus risperidone in the treatment of bipolar mania: improvement in manic and depressive symptoms and treatment adherence [abstract 15]. Presented at 156th American Psychiatric Association Annual Meeting. San Francisco, CA, May 17–22, 2003.

[37] Keck PE, McElroy SL, Strakowski SM, et al. Factors associated with maintenance antipsychotic treatment of patients with bipolar disorder. J Clin Psychiatry 1996;57(4):147–51.

[38] Miller DS, Yatham LN, Lam RW. Comparative efficacy of typical and atypical antipsychotics as add-on therapy to mood stabilizers in the treatment of acute mania. J Clin Psychiatry 2001;62(12):975–80.

[39] Zarate CA Jr. Antipsychotic drug side effect issues in bipolar manic patients. J Clin Psychiatry 2000;61(Suppl 8):52–61.

[40] Tohen M, Chengappa KNR, Suppes T, et al. Efficacy of olanzapine in combination with valproate or lithium in the treatment of mania in patients partially nonresponsive to valproate or lithium monotherapy. Arch Gen Psychiatry 2002;59(1):62–9.

[41] Sachs GS, Grossman F, Ghaemi SN, et al. Combination of a mood stabilizer with risperidone or haloperidol for treatment of acute mania: a double-blind, placebo-controlled comparison of efficacy and safety. Am J Psychiatry 2002;159(7):1146–54.

[42] Yatham LN, Grossman F, Augustyns I, et al. Mood stabilizer plus risperidone or placebo in the treatment of acute mania: international, double blind, randomized, controlled trial. Br J Psychiatry 2003; in press.

[43] Sachs G, Chengappa KNR, Suppes T, et al. Quetiapine with lithium or divalproex for the treatment of bipolar mania: a randomized, double-blind, placebo-controlled study. Bipolar Disord 2004;6(3):213–23.

[44] Yatham LN, Paulsson B, Mullen J, et al. Quetiapine versus placebo in combination with lithium or divalproex for the treatment of bipolar mania. J Clin Psychopharmacol 2004;24(6):599–606.

[45] DelBello MP, Schwiers ML, Rosenberg HL, et al. A double-blind, randomized, placebo-controlled study of quetiapine as adjunctive treatment for adolescent mania. J Am Acad Child Adolesc Psychiatry 2002;41(10):1216–23.

[46] Judd LL, Akiskal HS, Schettler PJ, et al. The long-term natural history of the weekly symptomatic status of bipolar I disorder. Arch Gen Psychiatry 2002;59(6):530–7.

[47] Tohen MF, Marneros A, Greil W, et al. Olanzapine versus lithium in relapse/recurrence prevention in bipolar disorder: a randomized double blind controlled 12 month clinical trial. Am J Psychiatry 2004, in press.

[48] Tohen M, Ketter TA, Zarate CA, et al. Olanzapine versus divalproex sodium for the treatment of acute mania and maintenance of remission: a 47-week study. Am J Psychiatry 2003;160(7):1263–71.

[49] Tohen M, Chengappa KNR, Suppes T, et al. Relapse prevention in bipolar I disorder: 18-month comparison of olanzapine plus mood stabiliser v. mood stabiliser alone. Br J Psychiatry 2004;184:337–45.

ELSEVIER
SAUNDERS

Psychiatr Clin N Am
28 (2005) 349–370

PSYCHIATRIC
CLINICS
OF NORTH AMERICA

Treatment of Bipolar Depression

Steven L. Dubovsky, MD[a,b,]*

[a]Department of Psychiatry, State University of New York at Buffalo,
462 Grider Street, Buffalo, NY 14215, USA
[b]University of Colorado School of Medicine, 4200 East Ninth Avenue,
Denver, CO 80262, USA

In contrast to unipolar depression, bipolar depression has not been the subject of many controlled trials. One likely reason for a paucity of empiric data about the treatment of this common and difficult problem is that people with bipolar mood disorders are more likely to drop out of research studies (as well as treatment) as their moods and motivation fluctuate. Bipolar disorder also has the highest rate of comorbidity with substance use disorder, which can complicate treatment and which usually disqualifies them from clinical trials. Most investigation of antidepressant regimens is sponsored by pharmaceutical manufacturers, who have little incentive to conduct expensive, multicenter trials with complicated patients who have a higher suicide risk and more comorbidity than patients with unipolar depression. Studies in patients with uniform depression are sufficient to obtain approval of a drug by the Food and Drug Administration (FDA). Patients with bipolar disorder who have been included in controlled clinical trials generally have had bipolar I depression or a low episode frequency; these patients do not necessarily resemble the average patient treated in clinical practice.

Methodologic shortcomings of many of the clinical trials that have been conducted in bipolar depression limit their application in clinical practice. Some studies lump together patients with bipolar and unipolar depression and then attempt to parse out treatment responses retrospectively. Without an a priori hypothesis about differential treatment responses, inferences drawn from this method can be used only to generate new hypotheses, not to prove a post hoc hypothesis. The same weakness applies to studies in which the study hypothesis is not supported, but a secondary outcome measure is found during retrospective data mining for changes in a favorable

* Department of Psychiatry, State University of New York at Buffalo, 462 Grider Street, Buffalo, NY 14215, USA.
  E-mail address: Dubovsky@buffalo.edu

direction. The few multicenter, controlled trials that have been published have relied on sample enrichment, in which only patients who respond during open treatment were assigned to a double-blind protocol, eliminating generalizability to unselected bipolar patients. Even in these samples, however, differences between patients were ignored, making it impossible to know which approaches are best for which patients. Bipolar depressed patients with frequent episodes may have a different treatment response than patients with fewer episodes, just as patients with agitation caused by mixed dysphoric hypomania or psychotic symptoms may do better with different treatments than patients with retarded bipolar depression.

In the absence of more definitive research, the treatment of bipolar depression is guided by clinical experience and expert opinion, and sometimes by marketing and popular trends, as much as it is by hard data. Considering the limitations of current knowledge is an essential component of the scientific practice of psychiatry.

Is bipolar depression a distinct type of depression?

Depressed mood is a nonspecific symptom that is not even limited to depressive disorders. Although bipolar and unipolar depression may respond acutely to some of the same treatments [1], they have distinct clinical and physiologic differences [2–4]. A century ago, Kraepelin [5] noted that bipolar depression is associated with lethargy, mental slowing, and hypersomnia, whereas unipolar depression is more frequently associated with agitation and insomnia, and that the risk of suicide is higher in bipolar depression. Although all mood disorders are recurrent, bipolar depression seems to recur more frequently. Psychotic symptoms are more common in bipolar depression, especially in younger patients, as is a family history of depression in consecutive generations. Biologic findings such as dexamethasone nonsuppression occur more frequently in bipolar depression, although it is not clear if this is a marker of bipolarity or of associated features such as severity or psychosis. On the other hand, markers that have been linked consistently to bipolar disorder, such as elevated free intracellular calcium ion concentration in blood platelets and lymphocytes (which occurs to a similar extent in mania and in bipolar depression), have not usually been observed in unipolar depression [6,7]. Such findings suggest that the treatment as well as the pathophysiology of bipolar depression might not be the same as for unipolar depression.

Bipolar disorder is not a unitary illness but a group of disorders with different courses and treatment responses [3]. In addition to categorical subgroups such as bipolar I and bipolar II disorder, conditions associated with a childhood onset, psychotic symptoms, a prominent affective family history, or comorbid substance abuse or contamination of the personality may be different disorders from adult-onset bipolar disorder in a patient without a family history of a mood disorder or significant comorbidity. Furthermore, features such as rapid or ultradian cycling may represent evolution of a mood disorder with a different pathophysiology and course than earlier stages of the disorder [8].

One subtype of bipolar depression that can be difficult to recognize is manifested by depression with mixed hypomanic symptoms. Mixed hypomanic symptoms in bipolar depression are often manifested by irritability, anxiety, or dysphoric overstimulation ("like crawling out of my skin"). Additional features may include insomnia (whereas hypersomnia is more common in uncomplicated bipolar depression), absence of anhedonia or increased sexual interest, profound irritability, and hypersensitivity to interpersonal and other forms of stimulation. The capacity to look substantially better than one feels may indicate an underlying element of elevated mood and energy. Although there are no studies of this issue, psychotic symptoms in bipolar depression, especially hallucinations, may also indicate significant activation mixed with depression. There is reason to think that antidepressants may exacerbate dysphoric hypomania mixed with depression, leading to a greater risk of mood destabilization than in uncomplicated bipolar depression.

Are antidepressants effective in bipolar depression?

Conventional wisdom holds that antidepressants are not as effective in bipolar depression as they are in unipolar depression. The few controlled studies that have been performed do not clearly support or refute this belief. In small, double-blind studies, the response rate of bipolar depression to imipramine was about 55% [9], which is not substantially different from response rates in unipolar depression. This impression received a little support from studies containing both unipolar and bipolar depressed patients in which response rates to tricyclic antidepressants (TCAs) were similar in both groups [2]. A review of controlled trials concluded that the combination of lithium and a TCA was no more effective than lithium monotherapy for acute treatment or prophylaxis of bipolar depression [10]. There are not enough studies containing a sufficient number of patients with bipolar depression to determine the true likelihood of response to TCAs, however. Similarly, data are insufficient to compare the efficacy of TCAs with second- and third-generation antidepressants in bipolar depression.

Newer antidepressants generally are believed to be as safe and possibly more effective for bipolar depression. A randomized trial that compared addition of paroxetine (n = 35), imipramine (n = 39), or placebo (n = 43) to ongoing lithium therapy in bipolar depression found no differences between the groups, however [11]. A double-blind study without a placebo control comparing bupropion to idozoxan found a response rate of about 50% for both medications [12].

Most other studies of the newer antidepressants in bipolar depression have involved open-label or single-blind addition of the antidepressant to mood stabilizers, with apparent efficacy of paroxetine, venlafaxine, fluoxetine, fluoxetine, citalopram, and nefazodone [2], although a randomized comparison of bupropion, venlafaxine, and sertraline in 64 patients reported a response rate less than 50% [13]. Similarly, a 6-week trial of random assignment of paroxetine or venlafaxine added to mood stabilizers for bipolar depression in 60 patients found response rates of 43% for paroxetine and 48% for venlafaxine [14], which were equivalent but not particularly impressive.

Experience in bipolar depression with the monoamine oxidase inhibitor antidepressants (MAOIs) goes back to the early 1970s. In an open-label study of patients with bipolar and unipolar anergic depression, three fourths of patients who had not responded to a TCA responded to tranylcypromine [15]. In subsequent double-blind studies, tranylcypromine was superior to placebo and to imipramine in the treatment of bipolar depression [16–18]. The reversible MAO-A inhibitor moclobemide (not available in the United States) has been found in controlled trials to be about as effective as imipramine but with fewer adverse effects in patients with bipolar or unipolar depression [2].

Stimulants have been known to have antidepressant properties for many years, and they are used regularly to treat depression in medically ill patients [19,20]. There are no controlled trials of these medications in bipolar depression, but an open study found methylphenidate to be well tolerated and rapidly effective [21]. Advantages of stimulants are that they can improve depression rapidly, and their effects may abate rapidly if adverse effects on mood develop.

A meta-analysis of 12 randomized trials of antidepressants in bipolar depression between 1980 and 2003 that lasted 4 to 10 weeks considered trials of distinctly different methodologies involving 1088 patients [22]. Two of these studies also included patients with unipolar depression. The majority of patients (75%) in the trials that were considered were treated concurrently with mood stabilizers or, in the case of the one olanzapine-fluoxetine trial discussed elsewhere in this article [23], olanzapine. Antidepressants were generally 1.2 to 2.9 times more likely to be associated with a response (either not defined, or at least 50% improvement in depression rating scale scores). In a tranylcypromine trial [16] that was included in the analysis, the antidepressant was 5.5 times as likely as a placebo to induce a response. The switch rate to mania was similar for antidepressants and placebo. As is true of the individual trials, interpretation of the findings is limited by the diverse methodologies, variable definitions of improvement, lack of prospective blind ratings of mania, and lack of consideration of antidepressant-induced manic syndromes less severe than mania. The risks of hypomania, cycle acceleration, and subsequent treatment resistance, as well as the possibility of antidepressant-induced recurrence of depression after 10 weeks of treatment, were not addressed in any of the studies included in the review.

Another view of antidepressant treatment of bipolar depression emerged in a careful chart review of antidepressant treatment of 37 patients with unipolar depression and 41 patients with bipolar depression, 55% of whom were also taking mood stabilizers [24]. Patients received one or more antidepressant trials. Antidepressants included selective serotonin reuptake inhibitors (SSRIs), venlafaxine, bupropion, nefazodone, mirtazepine, TCAs, MAOIs, and St. John's wort. Nonresponse to an antidepressant during the first 4 weeks of treatment was 1.6 times as likely in bipolar as in unipolar depression and was independent of coadministration of mood stabilizers. A new manic, hypomanic, or mixed episode occurred less than 8 weeks after starting an antidepressant in 49% of bipolar depressed patients (versus none of the unipolar depressed patients) and was more than four times as likely to occur without a mood stabilizer. Cycle acceleration (defined as two or more additional affective episodes beyond the number during a similar time before starting the antidepressant treatment) occurred in 26% of bipolar patients, and rapid cycling occurred in 32% of bipolar patients who took antidepressants for a year or more, a risk that was not reduced by concomitant use of mood stabilizers. Re-emergence of depression after 1 month or more of recovery was 3.4 times as likely in bipolar depression. No specific antidepressant was more likely than any other to induce manic/hypomanic switching, cycle acceleration, rapid cycling, or loss of response. In contrast, unipolar depressed patients who discontinued antidepressants were 4.7 times as likely as bipolar depressed patients to have a relapse of depression.

Epidemiologic studies suggest that antidepressants reduce suicidality in unipolar depression in younger [25], middle-aged [26], and older [27] individuals. Conversely, in a large naturalistic project, addition of antidepressants to mood stabilizers did not seem to be associated with a decreased incidence of suicidal ideation [28]. To the extent that antidepressants can aggravate mixed dysphoric hypomania in depressed patients, they could actually increase the risk of impulsive suicide by increasing overstimulation, impulsivity, and aggression as well as emotional discomfort. Juvenile-onset depression has a higher incidence of a bipolar outcome, and depression may be difficult to recognize because it begins before obvious hypomania. Therefore, it is possible that the recent observation of acutely increased new suicidal ideation or worsening of previous ideation in children and adolescents in clinical trials who took antidepressants versus those who took placebos [29] represents induction of dysphoric mixed states in patients whose bipolar depression was not identified at the start of the studies. In contrast, accumulating experience suggests that lithium reduces suicidal ideation and attempts separate from any antidepressant action [30].

Is lithium an antidepressant?

A number of controlled studies have demonstrated that lithium is effective in augmenting antidepressants, with greater response rates in bipolar than in unipolar depression [31]. In small, acute studies during the 1970s, lithium was found to be superior to placebo as monotherapy for bipolar depression [2], although some clinicians have found it to be less effective than antidepressants for this indication [2]. In an open study, the combination of lithium and carbamazepine was found to be effective in about half of patients with severe refractory bipolar depression [32]. Like all antimanic drugs, lithium seems to be more effective in preventing recurrences of depression than in treating it acutely and more likely to prevent recurrences of mania than recurrences of depression.

Anticonvulsants

In small, open-label studies and case reports, valproate, usually in combination with antidepressants or other antimanic drugs, has been reported to be useful in perhaps 30% to 50% of cases of bipolar depression [33,34]. A study of nine bipolar I patients with predominantly manic symptoms randomly assigned to take either divalproex or valproate (1–2 g/day) found reductions in the Hamilton Depression Rating Scale (HDRS) scores of 34 points with valproate and 10 points with divalproex [35]. Young Mania Rating Scale scores increased by 13 points with valproate, however, and they decreased by only 1 point in the divalproex group. The small number of subjects and the unexpected lack of an antimanic effect make any antidepressant action less reliable. In the absence of controlled research, it is impossible to know whether depressed patients who do benefit after addition of valproate have a true therapeutic response to valproate or its interaction with another medication, or whether they simply cycle out of depression. In clinical practice, valproate does not seem to be particularly effective as an antidepressant for most patients with bipolar or unipolar depression. On the other hand, an industry-sponsored, randomized, parallel-group, year-long study comparing valproate, lithium, and placebo in patients who recovered from a manic episode within 3 months found that patients taking valproate and an antidepressant were less likely to discontinue treatment because of depression than were patients taking placebo and an antidepressant [36]. The selection of patients for this maintenance study obviously favored valproate responders, because it excluded patients who did not improve with acute open treatment.

In contrast, carbamazepine may be somewhat more effective acutely for bipolar depression. In small, controlled studies, 50% to 68% of bipolar depressed patients have responded to carbamazepine [37,38]. Although data are not extensive, clinical experience suggests that carbamazepine can be effective acutely for bipolar depression, especially in combination with lithium.

Lamotrigine has been subjected to large, multicenter, industry-sponsored, controlled trials. In a 7-week double-blind study of 195 patients with bipolar I depression, both 50 and 200 mg/day of lamotrigine were equivalently superior to placebo in reducing Montgomery-Asberg Depression Rating Scale (MADRS) scores when observed cases were considered, but only the 200-mg dosage was superior to placebo in an intent-to-treat, last observation carried forward (LOCF) model [39]. About half the patients taking lamotrigine versus one fourth of those taking placebo had a response, and average MADRS scores decreased by about 50%; remission rates were not provided. In a 52-week continuation of this study, all patients were treated openly with lamotrigine, usually as an adjunct along with other medications deemed necessary by the treating physician [40]. Improvement of depression seemed to be sustained without mood destabilization.

In one of the two pivotal lamotrigine trials in bipolar depression [41], 349 recently depressed bipolar I patients were switched over 6 weeks from their previous treatment to lamotrigine for an 8- to 16-week open-label phase. Half of the sample (175 patients) stabilized on lamotrigine and was then randomly assigned for 18 months to lamotrigine, 50, 200, or 400 mg/day, lithium (serum level, 0.8–1.1 mM), or placebo. The 50-mg dosage of lamotrigine was ineffective, but the two higher dosages were both significantly more likely than placebo to lengthen the time to recurrence of depressive symptoms without any increase in manic symptoms over the 18 months. Thirty-six percent of lamotrigine patients versus 27% of placebo patients did not require an additional intervention for depression. In contrast, lithium, but not lamotrigine, was significantly better than placebo in lengthening the time to new intervention for a manic episode, without any increase in the risk of recurrence of depression. The generalizability of this finding is limited by the use of sample enrichment, which excluded half the initial sample and enrolled only patients in the double-blind phase who did well with open treatment with lamotrigine. Furthermore, patients were not acutely ill at the onset of the double-blind phase, and only bipolar I depression was studied.

The same methodologic concern applies to the other pivotal lamotrigine trial. In this study, currently or recently depressed bipolar I outpatients were treated openly with lamotrigine titrated up to 200 mg/day while other medications were withdrawn [42]. Of 966 patients enrolled in the study, less than half (463) completed the open-label phase. These patients were then randomly assigned to 50, 200, or 400 mg/day of lamotrigine, lithium (serum level, 0.8–1.1 mM), or placebo for 18 months. Lamotrigine and lithium both prolonged the time to intervention for any mood episode significantly more than placebo; the active treatments seemed to be equivalently effective for this purpose.

When data from the two latter studies were combined, lamotrigine did seem to be significantly more likely than placebo to lengthen the time to intervention for a new manic episode, leading to FDA approval as a maintenance treatment for bipolar disorder. For many illnesses, however, this kind of retrospective data mining from two studies with negative findings to produce one with a positive finding would not be considered compelling proof of efficacy, and the clinical implications of the new finding are not clear. Because the large, controlled trials considered only patients with bipolar I mood disorders who may not have had malignant courses, more information is necessary before clinicians can be confident that this medication is really a mood stabilizer.

Other new anticonvulsants have been thought to be useful for some depressed bipolar patients. Alone or in combination with standard mood stabilizers, gabapentin, which has not been found to be superior to placebo in patients with manic symptoms [43] or better than placebo or equal to lamotrigine in the treatment of manic and depressive symptoms [44], has improved bipolar depression in some small, open trials [45–47]. Topiramate, which has not been found to be a mood-stabilizing medication in controlled trials, has been thought to be useful for bipolar depression when combined with mood stabilizers [48]. Both topiramate (50–300 mg/day) and bupropion SR (100–400 mg/day) produced significant reductions of depressive symptoms in a single-blind 8-week trial in 36 outpatients with bipolar depression [49]. The rates of placebo response and spontaneous improvement would have been expected to be high in this group of mildly depressed patients, however. A chart review of 12 patients with bipolar depression for whom zonisamide was added to other medications noted that 50% responded, but improvement in Clinical Global Impressions (CGI) and Global Assessment of Functioning scores was not statistically significant [50]. There are no controlled studies of oxcarbazepine, levetiracetam, tiagabine, vigabactrin, and other anticonvulsants for bipolar depression.

Atypical antipsychotic medications

All atypical antipsychotics, with the possible exception of clozapine, have antidepressant properties, and even clozapine was helpful for a small number of patients with psychotic depression [51]. An 8-week study randomly assigned 542 patients with bipolar depression (358 of them bipolar I) to 300 or 600 mg/day of quetiapine or placebo [52]. In a LOCF analysis, mean MADRS scores decreased by 17 points with either dose of quetiapine and by 10 points with placebo; about one third of the placebo patients and half of the quetiapine patients responded.

The largest study of an antipsychotic drug in bipolar depression was an industry-sponsored study of olanzapine, which was designed primarily to demonstrate the efficacy of the combination of olanzapine and fluoxetine [23]. In this study, 833 patients with bipolar depression (duration 63–82 days) were randomly assigned for 8 weeks to placebo (n = 377), olanzapine, 5–20 mg (n = 370), or combinations of olanzapine and fluoxetine (doses of 6/25 mg, 6/50 mg, or 12/50 mg, respectively; n = 86). A major limitation was that half the active-treatment patients and two thirds of the placebo patients dropped out. For the remainder, both active treatments reduced depression scores more than placebo, with effect sizes of 0.32 for olanzapine and 0.68 for the combination of olanzapine and fluoxetine, mostly at higher doses of both medications. The effect size for olanzapine was low enough for it not to be an initial choice for treatment of bipolar depression. Given that the effect size for fluoxetine plus olanzapine was similar to the effect size for fluoxetine alone in unipolar depression, the combination did not seem to increase efficacy of the antidepressant. The conclusion that olanzapine prevented fluoxetine-induced mania cannot be supported by the short duration of the trial. Similarly, a post hoc analysis of data from two 3-week controlled trials of olanzapine in mania that found worsening of mania scores in 22% of olanzapine-treated patients and 38% of placebo patients [53] involved studies that were too short to justify the inference that atypical antipsychotic drugs with antidepressant properties do not induce mania. Additional weaknesses in these studies were that hypomania and mood cycling were not assessed, and the studies were not designed to address antipsychotic-induced mania. Conversely, case reports have been published of mania apparently associated with the institution of olanzapine treatment [54–56].

Electroconvulsive therapy

Electroconvulsive therapy (ECT) remains the most effective treatment for both unipolar and bipolar depression. In case series and naturalistic studies, ECT has been associated with equivalent efficacy in bipolar and unipolar depression and higher response rates than antidepressants in bipolar depression [57,58]. It has been suggested, but not proven, that the response to ECT may be more rapid in bipolar than in unipolar mood disorders, perhaps with a need for a lower stimulus intensity [59,60]. It has been suggested that the impression that bilateral ECT may be more effective than right unilateral ECT in bipolar depression could be the result of the shunting of current through the scalp with less than optimal unilateral placement [60].

Data on the efficacy of repetitive transcranial magnetic stimulation (rTMS) have been contradictory in unipolar depression, and most studies have not lasted more than a few weeks. In a study of bipolar depression, 23 patients were randomly assigned to daily left prefrontal rTMS or sham rTMS for 2 weeks [61]. There were no significant differences between the groups in improvement of depression. It is unknown whether longer treatment or a different placement might produce better results.

Dopamine agonists and other novel treatments

Open experience with piribedil [62] and bromocriptine [2] found rapid effectiveness for most of a small number of bipolar depressed patients but with a high likelihood of inducing mania. A chart review suggested that addition of pramipexole to other medications improved the response rate in bipolar as well as unipolar depression [63]. Such experience led to a 6-week randomized, controlled trial of pramipexole (mean dose, 1.7 mg) added to mood stabilizers in 22 outpatients with bipolar depression [64]. The primary outcome measure, reduction of HDRS scores by 50% or more, was achieved by two thirds of patients taking pramipexole and 20% taking placebo, but the difference just missed statistical significance because of the small sample ($P = 0.05$). There were significant differences between pramipexole and placebo in improvement of CGI scores, although these were secondary outcome measures. Only two pramipexole-treated patients and one placebo-treated patient achieved remission. As with the stimulants, the rapid onset and offset of action of dopaminergic medications could be beneficial and deserves further study, as does the possibly higher risk of inducing mania and mood cycling.

Mifepristone (RU-486), which is a progesterone receptor antagonist at low doses and a glucocorticoid receptor antagonist at higher doses, is currently under investigation as an adjunctive treatment for psychotic depression because dysregulated cortisol production is an essential component of this and other severe mood disorders. In a study of 20 patients with bipolar disorder, 19 of whom completed the trial, mifepristone or placebo was added to other treatments for 1 week, and patients were then crossed over to the other adjunct [65]. Follow-up 21 and 42 days later indicated cognitive improvement as well as reduction of HDRS scores by 5 points and MADRS scores by 6 points with mifepristone, versus no change with placebo. Continued treatment with a cortisol antagonist has been found to increase cortisol levels over time, making this an impractical chronic treatment. It is unclear whether any improvement with addition of mifepristone, which may indirectly antagonize dopaminergic transmission, would be sustained after it is discontinued.

Do antidepressants induce mania and rapid cycling?

Because rapid and ultradian cycling and other forms of deterioration of bipolar mood disorders are more likely to occur after an episode of mania or hypomania than after an episode of depression [66], the clinical implications of antidepressant-induced mania are important. From a scientific standpoint, however, it is difficult to determine the risk of antidepressant-induced mania or hypomania [67]. For one thing, there is no consensus about the definition of mania in response to an antidepressant. If mania develops for the first time a few weeks after starting use of an antidepressant, the likelihood seems greater that the antidepressant was to blame, but it is also possible that the association is coincidental. It would seem less likely that mania developing a year or more after starting use of an antidepressant was caused by that medication, but induction of mania, especially for the first time, might be a prolonged process in some patients. Most investigations of antidepressant-induced mania have considered only outright mania, but hypomania and subsyndromal hypomanic syndromes that can be difficult to recognize may have an equally important impact on the subsequent course of bipolar disorder. For patients who definitely develop mania or hypomania soon after starting use of an antidepressant for the first time, it is often not clear whether the antidepressant caused the change in polarity or whether the treatment with the antidepressant was started in an attempt to manage a deteriorating course that included the emergence of manic symptoms.

One of many unanswered questions is the relationship between antidepressant-induced mania or hypomania and the efficacy of the antidepressant in the first place. Clinical experience suggests that the likelihood that an antidepressant will cause hypomania or cycle acceleration is proportional to how effective it is for depression. If they are not immediately overstimulating, antidepressants seem less likely to affect mood adversely without first having an impact on depression. None of the few studies of antidepressant-induced mania has examined the correlation between the degree of improvement of depression in individual patients and the likelihood of subsequent deterioration of mood.

In a chart review of 51 bipolar disorder patients who had extensive life charting, 82% of patients developed mania while taking an antidepressant [67]. When a particularly stringent criterion for antidepressant-induced mania was used, it was determined that 35% of the patients developed a first episode of severe mania within 8 weeks of starting treatment with the antidepressant. Judging by the proximity of a first manic episode or cycle acceleration to starting treatment with an antidepressant, the investigators estimated that about 50% of the risk of these outcomes was attributable to antidepressants and the other half to spontaneous mood swings. An initial manic episode seemed to sensitize patients to subsequent manic episodes and rapid cycling. It was not clear, on the other hand, that mood stabilizers were able to prevent these outcomes.

In a longitudinal study, Coryell et al [68] concluded that the use of TCAs and MAOIs did not seem to predate rapid cycling predictably when the presence of depression was controlled. As Wehr [69] pointed out, however, this interpretation is limited by the authors' simply correlating use of antidepressants at the time of entry into their study with rapid cycling during the following year. They did not examine whether treatment with antidepressants was initiated or withdrawn during the study period. Another flaw was that the prevalence of rapid cycling declined from 19% to 5% over 1 year of follow-up, but the investigators did not determine whether this change was associated with withdrawing antidepressants. In an earlier prospective study of a group of patients with rapid cycling, cycling was more severe while patients were taking antidepressants (mostly TCAs) despite the concurrent use of mood stabilizers; the duration of cycling decreased when antidepressants were withdrawn [70].

There are no direct comparisons of antidepressants with a placebo arm to control for spontaneous switch rates that were undertaken with the a priori intent of demonstrating differences in induction of mania or hypomania. As a result, any impressions of a differential likelihood of mania induction with different antidepressants are limited. The TCAs traditionally are considered more likely than the newer antidepressants to induce mania, but there is a little evidence from clinical trials that switch rates are distinctly higher for TCAs than for SSRIs and bupropion [2]. These studies, however, were not designed to investigate differential switch rates, so the most that can be said is that this is a hypothesis worth investigating in a controlled study. Comparisons of switch rates in TCA clinical trials with trials of new antidepressants are probably limited by the methodologies of these studies, most of which were industry supported and were designed to demonstrate efficacy and safety in unipolar, not bipolar, depression. Bipolar disorder is an exclusion criterion in these trials, but the ability of investigators to apply this criterion has improved considerably with greater awareness of the polymorphic manifestations of bipolar illness. One consequence of this change is that fewer depressed patients in trials of newer antidepressants are as likely to have been bipolar and therefore to develop a manic switch than was true in the earlier TCA trials.

Reports of different switch rates with different classes of antidepressants in bipolar depression [28] are not particularly reliable because they rely on data from individual studies with different methodologies. Conclusions drawn from post hoc analysis of data obtained for other purposes cannot be used to prove a hypothesis about antidepressant-induced mania. No prospective study has been conducted to compare switch rates with different antidepressants at equivalent doses in matched patients.

A subset of 37 patients in a randomized study of fluoxetine monotherapy took open-label fluoxetine (20 mg/day) for up to 8 weeks [71]. During this time, three patients developed hypomania, and a fourth cycled into a more severe depression, leading the authors to conclude that the switch rate was low. Fluoxetine was used as monotherapy in an open trial for depression in 16 patients with well-described bipolar II disorder [72]. Over 3 years of variable levels of observation, patients did not develop mania or hypomania. The mood disorder also did not deteriorate in open experience with another small sample of patients with bipolar II depression treated with venlafaxine alone [73]. The lack of a control, independent ratings, random selection, or an a priori hypothesis makes these kinds of reports at best suggestive that a subgroup of bipolar depressed patients is able to tolerate antidepressants without a mood stabilizer. It is not possible to identify such patients in advance, however.

Conventional wisdom holds that bupropion is less likely to induce mania than other antidepressants. This impression is derived from small initial studies in which the switch rate seemed to be lower than that reported with other antidepressants, but there has not been a prospective direct comparison between bupropion and other antidepressants in which the primary goal was to evaluate the new incidence of hypomania or mania. During open observation, more than 50% of 11 patients with a history of developing mania with other antidepressants also had a manic switch on bupropion even though they were also taking mood stabilizers [74].

Most publications on the topic suggest that MAOIs are more likely to induce mania than other antidepressant classes [2]. This impression may based in part be on diagnostic trends in the decade in which MAOI trials were conducted compared with later antidepressant trials. In addition, because treatment-emergent mania is documented poorly in most of these studies, it remains to be determined whether any apparently higher rate of mania simply reflects the more-activating MAOIs causing more insomnia, nervousness, and dysphoria. An analysis of 155 antidepressant trials in 41 depressed patients found no difference in the likelihood of mania induction between bupropion, SSRIs, TCAs, MAOIs, and other new antidepressants [75]. The risk of mania was twice as high in patients who were not also taking mood stabilizers.

Because rapid cycling and other forms of deterioration of mood in bipolar mood disorders often follow a manic episode, a major concern about antidepressant-induced mania is that it may be followed by cycle acceleration and treatment resistance [28]. About 20% of patients with rapid cycling in the *Diagnostic and Statistical Manual-IV* (DSM-IV) field trials seemed to have been precipitated by antidepressants [76]. In a population of treatment-refractory patients with ultradian cycling, mood stabilizers were not particularly effective, but withdrawing antidepressants improved outcome [77].

In the absence of prospective, controlled trials in different categories of patients, it also is not known which bipolar patients are more likely to develop mood destabilization with antidepressants. A chart review of 169 patients with bipolar I or bipolar II disorder suggested that the former were more likely to develop antidepressant-induced mania [78]. Retrospective analyses of data from a variety of naturalistic settings suggest that risk factors include family history of bipolar disorder, early onset of the mood disorder, comorbid substance use disorder, history of rapid cycling or antidepressant-induced mania with other medications, and multiple antidepressant trials [28]. Patients who report that an antidepressant worked within hours to days may be more likely to have a bipolar mood disorder and to develop treatment resistance [79]. A chart review of 158 inpatients with bipolar I depression suggested that when patients in whom depression was mixed with hypomanic symptoms such as racing thoughts, logorrhea, aggression, irritability, distractibility, and increased drive were more likely to develop antidepressant-induced manic switches [80].

Continuation of antidepressants

When an antidepressant is clearly effective for bipolar depression, an important clinical controversy revolves around whether continuation of the antidepressant may eventually destabilize mood. This problem may be manifested as mania or hypomania, often following by cycling into another depressive episode. A subtler outcome involves the antidepressant's first increasing the likelihood of remission of depression but then increasing the likelihood of recurrence. As a result, the patient has a robust antidepressant response (which often is very rapid), followed by what seems to be relapse but actually represents a new episode provoked by the antidepressant. A change in the antidepressant leads to another remission, followed by another recurrence. This outcome is difficult to study because there is no clear consensus about how long after starting treatment with an anti-depressant hypomania or a recurrence of depression should be attributed to that medication rather than to the natural course of the illness, and the problem of recurrences of depression driven by antidepressants has not been studied in controlled trials. Extended, prospective, random assignment studies of patients with similar subtypes of bipolar depression might answer this question, but such studies are ethically and practically problematic. In the meantime, the little evidence that has accumulated suggests that mood stabilizers do not necessarily prevent destabilization of mood by anti-depressants [67,77].

The National Institute of Mental Health collaborative study on mainte-nance treatment in mood disorders seemed to find that patients did not develop rapid cycling despite taking antidepressants chronically along with mood stabilizers [77]. Patients were entered into the study only if their moods were stable after open treatment with an antidepressant, however, and 46% of patients who began antidepressant therapy did not meet this criterion. A more accurate conclusion would be that approximately half of patients who begin taking antidepressants for bipolar depression do not improve or get worse, whereas the same number may be able to tolerate these medications.

A similar comment applies to a well-publicized study of 1078 patients with bipolar disorder in the Stanley Foundation network during a naturalistic study of treatment outcome [81]. Of this group, 549 received an antidepressant for bipolar depression in addition to ongoing treatment with a mood stabilizer. Only 189 patients continued taking the antidepressant for at least 6 weeks (reasons for discontinuing the antidepressant were not given), and 84 of these responded. The 84 antidepressant responders were divided into those who took the medication for 6 months or less and those who took the antidepressant for more than 6 months. The former group (n = 43) took the antidepressant for an average of 74 days, and the latter (n = 41) for 484 days. The risk of depressive relapse was about four times higher in the group that discontinued the antidepressant in a little over 2 months. The risk of manic relapse was about 18% in both groups. The authors concluded that early antidepressant discontinuation increases the risk of depressive relapse, whereas continuing antidepressants does not increase the risk of mania.

Another interpretation of the data is that only 15% of the patients who begin taking an antidepressant or 44% of those who can stay on an antidepressant for at least 6 weeks respond to the medication; at best, the latter rate is similar to the placebo response rate in major depression. In addition, antidepressants may have been withdrawn early because patients were relapsing, or rapid withdrawal of the antidepressant could have caused rebound depression. A major methodologic problem in addition to the open method was the use of a single global rating by the primary clinician (CGI-Bipolar), not distinguishing whether the patient was euthymic, manic, or depressed. Hypomania, rapid cycling, and subsyndromal affective dysregulation were not considered. Equally important, the rate of manic recurrence was substantially lower in the entire group than has been reported in other studies from the Stanley Foundation subjects. The statistical method has been criticized also [82]. The only definitive conclusion that can be drawn from this study that is consistent with other work is that there is a small group of bipolar depressed patients whose moods remain stable for a year or more on the combination of an antidepressant and a mood stabilizer. It is not yet possible to distinguish in advance these patients from the majority who do not respond to antidepressants or who get worse while taking them.

Mixed hypomanic symptoms might predispose a patient to deterioration of mood with antidepressants. In a study of 40 symptomatic patients with DSM-IV rapid cycling, depression accompanied by mixed manic symptoms seemed to be associated with a more severe illness that was exacerbated by use of antidepressants [83]. Patients with major depression with mixed manic features were less likely to receive a mood stabilizer than were patients without such features.

Recommendations

Although some patients may do well with antidepressants alone, there are no data to indicate how to identify these patients in advance, and only a minority of expert consensus panel respondents recommends use of an antidepressant without a mood stabilizer in bipolar depression [28]. Otherwise, it seems prudent to begin treatment for bipolar depression with a mood-stabilizing medication. Fig. 1 describes an algorithm for subsequent treatment. Because retrospective recall of mood may be colored by how the patient feels at the moment, keeping a daily mood chart can facilitate assessment of the response to each intervention.

Based on the limited available data, lithium or carbamazepine may be better initial choices for bipolar depression than valproate. Although lamotrigine may be appropriate as maintenance therapy for some patients with recent bipolar I depression, there are no controlled data to support the use of this medication as a first-line monotherapy for other forms of bipolar depression. There is no evidence that it is an antimanic drug other than tenuous conclusions drawn from unjustified combinations of data from studies done for other purposes. Nevertheless, most practice guidelines consider lamotrigine to be a first-line treatment for bipolar depression in general. A recent consensus conference recommended lamotrigine

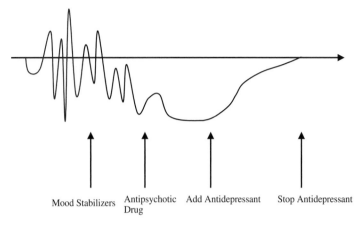

Mood Stabilizers Antipsychotic Add Antidepressant Stop Antidepressant
                  Drug

Fig. 1. Treatment of bipolar depression.

monotherapy for mild to moderate bipolar depression and a combination of
lamotrigine and lithium or an atypical antipsychotic was preferred for more
severe depression [84]. Lamotrigine can be useful at times, but at other
times, contrary to published data in patients with a low frequency of manic
recurrence, it rapidly induces hypomania. Short-term studies with extremely
high dropout rates do not support the use of an olanzapine-fluoxetine
combination as first-line treatment for bipolar depression given other
options that are available as initial therapies [84].

   The next step depends on whether there are any mixed hypomanic
symptoms or dramatic fluctuations of mood suggestive of mood cycling. It
might seem intuitively obvious that both poles of a mixed bipolar depression
can be easily treated at the same time, but in some cases the antidepressant
may stimulate more activation or may increase the likelihood of depressive
recurrence in the presence of mixed hypomania, and it is not yet known
which patients will be susceptible to this problem. Although there are no
definitive studies of this question, long-term outcomes may be better if mixed
hypomania is eliminated before the depression is treated. Adding a second
mood stabilizer may achieve this goal. If not, additional mood stabilizers
might be added. Valproate can be a useful addition, as can some of the newer
anticonvulsants discussed elsewhere in this issue. A calcium-channel blocker
might also be considered.

   Antipsychotic medications can be useful in suppressing mixed dysphoric
hypomania in bipolar depression, and atypical antipsychotics generally are
recommended rather than neuroleptics, which have been associated with
worsening depression [84]. Doses used in pivotal trials in bipolar I depression
may not apply to patients with more complex presentations of depression.
Because the antidepressant properties of atypical antipsychotics may be dose
dependent [85], lower doses are preferable in treating mixed states, as least
initially.

Sometimes, slow adjustment of the mood-stabilizing regimen will stabilize mood in a euthymic range, especially if affective symptoms have been fluctuating substantially. At least as often in clinical practice, however, mood stabilizers are more rapidly effective against mixed hypomanic symptoms than against depression. In this case, symptoms such as insomnia, agitation, irritability, distractibility, and psychotic symptoms remit, but patients feel more consistently sluggish or depressed. An antidepressant may be more effective and less likely to induce mood cycling in this state of less complicated bipolar depression. The traditional choice of bupropion as an initial antidepressant is reasonable, but the evidence that this medication really is safer in bipolar depression is equivocal, and most other antidepressants are equally appropriate choices. Despite mixed data on the greater likelihood of mania induction with TCAs, these medications are later choices in the treatment of depression. Lamotrigine may be one of the better initial choices for bipolar depression. A stimulant could also be considered. The MAOIs still may be among the more effective treatments for bipolar depression. As mentioned earlier, atypical antipsychotic drugs can be used adjunctively to treat bipolar depression.

Another option for the treatment of bipolar depression is artificial bright light. There is, of course, a substantial literature on this treatment for seasonal affective disorder, in which bipolar depression is over-represented, but not much research has been conducted in other forms of bipolar disorder. An advantage of bright light is that the dose can be adjusted very precisely to a duration that improves depression but stays below the threshold for induction of mania and cycle acceleration. Bright light is most appropriate for bipolar depression with a seasonal variation, but it sometimes is effective for nonseasonal bipolar depression, especially if the depression is accompanied by hypersomnia or a phase reversal of the sleep-wake cycle. In the latter case, morning bright light may improve the sleep disorder as well as the depression.

All these changes should be made gradually in outpatients. Rapid increases in doses of mood stabilizers may increase the likelihood that they will suppress agitation and related hypomanic symptoms before they treat depression. Rapid reductions of antidepressant doses may increase the risk of rebound depression, which can create the mistaken impression that antidepressant withdrawal is causing relapse.

Because it is not yet possible to determine in advance which patients may tolerate long-term treatment with an antidepressant, it is prudent to attempt to withdraw the antidepressant very slowly once the depression has remitted completely. The decision to withdraw the antidepressant can be a complex judgment, because patients may feel significantly better without feeling well, and relapse is more likely in the presence of any residual symptoms. Mood stabilizers should be continued indefinitely for most patients.

Most studies of psychotherapy for depression exclude patients with bipolar depression or find lower response rates in that condition.

Nevertheless, well-documented treatments such as cognitive behavior therapy and interpersonal therapy should be considered [84]. Family-focused therapy and interpersonal and social rhythms therapy have been found to be useful as maintenance therapies in bipolar disorder and have been recommended for bipolar depression [84]. It is rare that people with bipolar depression, who experience considerable suffering, do not have psychologic and family issues that require rigorous attention.

There are no studies of refractory bipolar depression. ECT is an obvious intervention in such cases, but most mood stabilizers except for calcium-channel blockers should be withdrawn before this treatment. If repeated antidepressant trials have been unsuccessful, or if the patient has responded but then relapsed, the mood chart should be reviewed carefully to determine whether subtle mood cycling or dysphoric hypomania is present that might be exacerbated rather than helped by the antidepressant.

The treatment of bipolar depression requires substantial expertise in the art as well as the science of psychiatry. Because mixed and highly recurrent bipolar depression is more complex physiologically than simpler forms of bipolar disorder, combinations of treatments are often necessary. Informed consent includes discussing the limitations of scientific knowledge about this condition and underscoring the importance of close follow-up to determine the best treatment for an individual patient. With careful attention to subtle and subsyndromal symptoms and associated psychologic and family issues, the outcome of treatment can be rewarding.

References

[1] Abrams R, Taylor MA. A comparison of unipolar and bipolar depressive illness. Am J Psychiatry 1980;137:1084–7.
[2] Silverstone PH, Silverstone T. A review of acute treatments for bipolar depression. Int Clin Psychopharmacol 2004;19:113–24.
[3] Dubovsky SL, Dubovsky AN. Concise guide to mood disorders. Washington (DC): American Psychiatric Press; 2002.
[4] Kessing LV, Hansen M, Andersen PK. Course of illness in depressive and bipolar disorders. Br J Psychiatry 2004;185:372–7.
[5] Ey H. Kraepelin centenary; the problem of endogenous psychoses in the German School of psychiatry. Evol Psychiatry (Paris) 1956;4:951–8. [In French].
[6] Dubovsky SL, Lee C, Christiano J. Elevated intracellular calcium ion concentration in bipolar depression. Biol Psychiatry 1991;29:441–50.
[7] Dubovsky SL, Murphy J, Thomas M, et al. Abnormal intracellular calcium ion concentration in platelets and lymphocytes of bipolar patients. Am J Psychiatry 1992;149:118–120.
[8] Dubovsky SL. Current approaches to the treatment of rapid cycling bipolar disease. Curr Psychiatry Rep 2001;3:451–62.
[9] Srisurapanont ML, Sachs G, Bowden C, et al. Double-blind, placebo controlled comparison of imipramine and paroxetine in the treatment.
[10] Ghaemi SN, Lenox MS, Baldessarini RJ. Effectiveness and safety of long-term anti-depressanttreatment in bipolar disorder. J Clin Psychiatry 2001;62:565–9.

[11] Nemeroff CB, Evans DL, Gyulai L, et al. Double-blind, placebo controlled comparison of imipramine and paroxetine in the treatment of bipolar depression. Am J Psychiatry 2001; 158:906–12.

[12] Grossman F, Potter WZ, Brown EA, et al. A double-blind study comparing idazoxan and bupropion in bipolar depressed patients. J Psychiatr Res 1999;7:171–83.

[13] Post RM, Altshuler L, Frye M, et al. Rate of switch in bipolar patients prospectively treated with second generation antidepressants as augmentation to mood stabilizers. Bipolar Disord 2001;3:259–65.

[14] Vieta E, Martinez-Aran A, Goikolea J, et al. A randomized trial comparing paroxetine and venlafaxine in the treatment of bipolar depressed patients taking mood stabilizers. J Clin Psychiatry 2002;63:508–12.

[15] Himmelhoch JM, Detre T, Kupfer DJ, et al. Treatment of previously intractable depression with tranylcypromine and lithium. J Nerv Ment Dis 1972;155:216–20.

[16] Himmelhoch JM, Fuchs C, Symons BJ. A double-blind study of tranylcypromine treatment of major anergic depression. J Nerv Ment Dis 1982;170:628–34.

[17] Himmelhoch JM, Thase ME, Mallinger AG, et al. Tranylcypromine versus imipramine in anergic bipolar depression. Am J Psychiatry 1991;148:910–6.

[18] Thase ME, Mallinger AG, McKnight D, et al. Treatment of imipramine-resistant recurrent depression, IV: a double-blind crossover study of tranylcypromine for anergic bipolar depression. Am J Psychiatry 1992;149:195–8.

[19] Wagner GJ, Rabkin R. Effects of dextroamphetamine on depression and fatigue in men with HIV: a double-blind, placebo-controlled trial. J Clin Psychiatry 2000;61:436–40.

[20] Warneke L. Psychostimulants in psychiatry [review]. Can J Psychiatry 1990;35(1):3–10.

[21] El-Mallakh RS. An open study of methylphenidate in bipolar depression. Bipolar Disord 2000;2:56–9.

[22] Gijsman HJ, Geddes J, Rendell J, et al. Antidepressants for bipolar depression: a systematic review of randomized, controlled trials. Am J Psychiatry 2004;161:1537–47.

[23] Tohen M, Vieta E, Calabrese JR, et al. Efficacy of olanzapine and olanzapine-fluoxetine combination in the treatment of bipolar I depression. Arch Gen Psychiatry 2003;60: 1079–88.

[24] Ghaemi SN, Rosenquist KJ, Ko JY, et al. Antidepressant treatment in bipolar versus unipolar depression. Am J Psychiatry 2004;161:163–5.

[25] Olfson M, Shaffer D, Marcus SC, et al. Relationship between antidepressant medication treatment and suicide in adolescents. Arch Gen Psychiatry 2003;60:978–82.

[26] Grunebaum MF, Ellis SP, Li S, et al. Antidepressants and suicide risk in the United States, 1985–1999. J Clin Psychiatry 2004;65:1456–62.

[27] Hall W, Mant PB, Rendle VA, et al. Association between antidepressant prescribing and suicide in Australia, 1991–2000: trend analysis. BMJ 2003;326:1–5.

[28] Goldberg J. When do antidepressants worsen the course of bipolar disorder? J Psychiatr Pract 2003;9:181–94.

[29] United States Food and Drug Administration (FDA). Worsening depression and suicidality in patients being treated with antidepressant medications FDA Public Health Advisory, March 22, 2004.

[30] Muller-Oerlinghausen B. Arguments for the specificity of the antisuicidal effect of lithium. Eur Arch Psychiatry Clin Neurosci 2001;251(Suppl2):72–5.

[31] Price LH, Charney DS, Heninger GR. Variability of response to lithium augmentation in refractory depression. Am J Psychiatry 1986;143:1387–92.

[32] Kramlinger KG, Post RM. The addition of lithium to carbamazepine: antidepressant efficacy in treatment-resistant depression. Arch Gen Psychiatry 1989;46:794–800.

[33] Calabrese JR, Delucchi GA. Spectrum of efficacy of valproate in 55 patients with rapid cycling bipolar disorder. Am J Psychiatry 1990;147:431–4.

[34] McElroy SL, Keck PE. Treatment guidelines for valproate in bipolar and schizoaffective disorders. Can J Psychiatry 1993;38(Suppl2):S31–8.

[35] Kablinger AS, Czerwinski WP, Minagar A. Divalproex versus valproate in patients with bipolar disorder. J Clin Psychopharmacol 2004;24:231–2.

[36] Gyulai L, Bowden C, McElroy SL, et al. Maintenance efficacy of divalproex in the prevention of bipolar depression. Neuropsychopharmacology 2003;28:1374–82.

[37] Post RM, Uhde TW, Roy-Byrne PP, et al. Antidepressant effects of carbamazepine. Am J Psychiatry 1986;143:29–34.

[38] Brambilla P, Barale F, Soares JC. Perspectives on the use of anticonvulsants in the treatment of bipolar disorder. Int J Neuropsychopharmacol 2001;4:421–46.

[39] Calabrese JR, Bowden CL, Sachs GS, et al. A double-blind placebo-controlled study of lamotrigine monotherapy in outpatients with bipolar I depression. Lamictal 602 Study Group. J Clin Psychiaty 1999;60:79–88.

[40] McElroy SL, Zarate CA, Cookson J, et al. A 52-week, open-label continuation study of lamotrigine in the treatment of bipolar depression. J Clin Psychiatry 2004;65:204–10.

[41] Bowden C, Calabrese JR, Sachs G, et al. A placebo-controlled 18-month trial of lamotrigine and lithium maintenance treatment in recently manic or hypomanic patients with bipolar I disorder. Arch Gen Psychiatry 2003;60:392–400.

[42] Calabrese JR, Bowden C, Sachs G, et al. A placebo-controlled 18-month trial of lamotrigine and lithium maintenance treatment in recently depressed patients with bipolar I disorder. J Clin Psychiatry 2003;64:1013–24.

[43] Pande AC, Crockatt JG, Janney CA, et al. Gabapentin in bipolar disorder: a placebo-controlled trial of adjunctive therapy. Gabapentin Bipolar Disorder Study Group. Bipolar Disord 2000;2(3 Pt 2):249–55.

[44] Frye MA, Ketter TA, Kimbrell TA, et al. A placebo-controlled study of lamotrigine and gabapentin monotherapy in refractory mood disorders. J Clin Psychopharmacol 2000;20:607–14.

[45] Young LT, Robb J, Patelis-Siotis I, et al. Acute treatment of bipolar depression with gabapentin. Biol Psychiatry 1997;42:851–3.

[46] Wang PW, Santosa C, Schumacher M, et al. Gabapentin augmentation therapy in bipolar depression. Bipolar Disord 2002;4:296–301.

[47] Sokolski KN, Green C, Maris DE, et al. Gabapentin as an adjunct to standard mood stabilizers in outpatients with mixed bipolar symptomatology. Ann Clin Psychiatry 1999;11:217–22.

[48] Yatham LN, Calabrese JR, Kusumaker V. Bipolar depression: treatment options. Can J Psychiatry 2003;42(suppl 2):87S–91S.

[49] McIntyre R, Mancini DA, McCann S, et al. Topiramate versus bupropion SR when added to mood stabilizer for the depressive phase of bipolar disorder: a preliminary single-blind study. Bipolar Disord 2002;4:207–13.

[50] Baldassano CF, Ghaemi SN, Chang A, et al. Acute treatment of bipolar depression with adjunctive zonisamide: a retrospective chart review. Bipolar Disord 2004;6:432–4.

[51] Rothschild AJ. Management of psychotic, treatment-resistant depression. Psychiatr Clin N Am 1996;19(2):237–52.

[52] Calabrese JR. Controlled study of quetiapine for bipolar disorder. Presented at The American Psychiatric Association Meeting, New York, NY, May 1–6, 2004.

[53] Baker R, Milton D, Stauffer VL, et al. Placebo-controlled trials do not find association of olanzapine with exacerbation of bipolar mania. J Affect Disord 2003;73:147–53.

[54] Benazzi F. Olanzapine-induced psychotic mania in bipolar schizo-affective disorder [letter]. Eur Psychiatry 1999;14:410–1.

[55] Borysewicz K, Borysewicz W. A case of mania following olanzapine administration. Psychiatr Pol 2000;34:299–306.

[56] Fitz-Gerald MJ, Pinkofsky HB, Brannon G, et al. Olanzapine-induced mania [letter]. Am J Psychiatry 1999;156:1114.

[57] Black DW, Winokur G, Nasrallah HA. The treatment of depression: electroconvulsive therapy versus antidepressants: a naturalistic evaluation of 1495 patients. Compr Psychiatry 1987;28:169–82.

[58] Grunhaus L, Schreiber S, Dolberg O, et al. Response to ECT in major depression: are there differences between unipolar and bipolar depression? Bipolar Disord 2002;4(Suppl 1): 91–3.

[59] Daly JJ, Prudic J, Devanand DP, et al. ECT in bipolar and unipolar depression: differences in speed of response. Bipolar Disord 2001;3:95–104.

[60] Mukherjee S, Sackeim HA, Schnur DB. Electroconvulsive therapy of acute manic episodes: a review of 50 years' experience. Am J Psychiatry 1994;151:169–76.

[61] Nahas Z, Kozel FA, Li X, et al. Left prefrontal transcranial magnetic stimulation (TMS) treatment of depression in bipolar affective disorder: a pilot study of acute safety or efficacy. Bipolar Disord 2003;5:40–7.

[62] Post RM, Gerner RH, Carman JS, et al. Effects of a dopamine agonist pribedil in depressed patients; relationship of pretreatment homovanillic acid to antidepressant response. Arch Gen Psychiatry 1978;35:609–15.

[63] Sporn J, Ghaemi SN, Sambur MR, et al. Pramipexole augmentation in the treatment of unipolar and bipolar depression: a retrospective chart review. Ann Clin Psychiatry 2000;12: 137–40.

[64] Goldberg J, Burdick KE, Endick CJ. Preliminary randomized, double-blind, placebo-controlled trial of pramipexole added to mood stabilizers for treatment-resistant bipolar depression. Am J Psychiatry 2004;161:564–6.

[65] Young A, Gallagher P, Watson S, et al. Improvements in neurocognitive function and mood following adjunctive treatment with mifepristone (RU-486) in bipolar disorder. Neuropsychopharmacology 2004;29:1538–45.

[66] Post RM, Roy-Byrne PP, Uhde TW. Graphic representation of the life course of illness in patients with affective disorder. Am J Psychiatry 1988;145:844–8.

[67] Altshuler LL, Post RM, Leverich GS, et al. Antidepressant-induced mania and cycle acceleration: a controversy revisited. Am J Psychiatry 1995;152(8):1130–8.

[68] Coryell W, Endicott J, Keller M. Rapidly cycling affective disorder: demographics, diagnosis, family history and course. Arch Gen Psychiatry 1992;49:126–31.

[69] Wehr TA. Can antidepressants induce rapid cycling? Arch Gen Psychiatry 1993;50(6):495–6.

[70] Wehr T, Sack D, Rosenthal N, et al. Rapid cycling affective disorder: contributing factors and treatment responses in 51 patients. Am J Psychiatry 1988;145:179–84.

[71] Amsterdam JD, Shults J, Brunswick DJ, et al. Short-term fluoxetine monotherapy for bipolar type II or bipolar NOS major depression–low manic switch rate. Bipolar Disord 2004;6:75–81.

[72] Simpson SG, DePaulo JR. Fluoxetine treatment of bipolar II depression. J Clin Psychopharmacol 1991;11:52–4.

[73] Amsterdam JD, Garcia-Espana F. Venlafaxine monotherapy in women with bipolar II and unipolar major depression. J Affect Disord 2000;59:225–9.

[74] Fogelson DL, Bystritsky A, Pasnau R. Buproprion in the treatment of bipolar disorders: the same old story. J Clin Psychiatry 1992;53:443–6.

[75] Goldberg J, Ernst CL. Features associated with the delayed initiation of mood stabilizers at illness onset in bipolar disorder. J Clin Psychiatry 2002;63:985–91.

[76] Bauer M, Calabrese JR, Dunner DL. Multisite data reanalysis of the validity of rapid cycling as a course modifier for bipolar disorder in DSM-IV. Am J Psychiatry 1994;151:506–15.

[77] Prien RF, Kupfer DJ, Mansky PA. Drug therapy in the prevention of recurrences in unipolar and bipolar affective disorders: report of the NIMH Collaborative Study Group comparing lithium carbonate, imipramine, and a lithium carbonate-imipramine combination. Arch Gen Psychiatry 1984;41:1096–104.

[78] Serretti A, Artioli P, Zanardi R, et al. Clinical features of antidepressant associated manic and hypomanic switches in bipolar disorder. Prog Neuropsychopharmacol Biol Psychiatry 2003;27:751–7.

[79] Piver A. Ultrarapid response to an antidepressant: a clue to bipolarity? Can J Psychiatry 2003;48:427–8.

[80] Bottlender R, Sato T, Kleindiest N, et al. Mixed depressive features predict a maniform switch during rx of depression in bipolar I disorder. J Affect Disord 2004;78:149–52.

[81] Altshuler L, Suppes T, Black D, et al. Impact of antidepressant discontinuation after acute bipolar depression remission on rates of depressive relapse at 1-year follow-up. Am J Psychiatry 2003;160:1252–62.

[82] Soldani F, Ghaemi SN, Tondo L, et al. Relapse after antidepressant discontinuation [letter]. Am J Psychiatry 2004;161:1312–3.

[83] Goldberg JF, Wankmuller MM, Sutherland KH. Depression with versus without manic features in rapid-cycling bipolar disorder. J Nerv Ment Dis 2004;192:602–6.

[84] Keck PE, Perlis RH, Otto MW, et al. Treatment of bipolar disorder 2004. Postgrad Med 2004; special report:1–120.

[85] Tollefson GD, Beasley CM Jr, Tran PV, et al. Olanzapine versus haloperidol in the treatment of schizophrenia and schizoaffective and schizophreniform disorders: results of an international collaborative trial. Am J Psychiatry 1997;154(4):457–65.

ELSEVIER
SAUNDERS

Psychiatr Clin N Am
28 (2005) 371–384

PSYCHIATRIC
CLINICS
OF NORTH AMERICA

Psychosocial Treatments for Bipolar Disorders

Jan Scott, MD, FRCPsych[a,*],
Francesc Colom, D Clin Psych, PhD[a,b]

[a]Division of Psychological Medicine, Institute of Psychiatry, P.O. Box 96,
De Crespigny Park, Denmark Hill, London SE5 8AF, UK
[b]Department of Psychiatry, Bipolar Disorders Program, Stanley Centre for Bipolar
Disorders Research, Villarroel 170, Barcelona 08036, Spain

The increased acceptance of stress-vulnerability models of severe mental disorders and of brief evidence-based psychologic treatments for these disorders has led to increased interest in the role of psychotherapies in treating bipolar disorders (BP). This article discusses the rationale for the use of psychologic treatments as an adjunct to usual treatment and reviews the randomized, controlled trials of specific therapy models, such as group psychoeducation and individual cognitive therapy, that tackle a spectrum of complex psychologic and social problems associated with BP. These treatment-outcome studies generally support the efficacy of adjunctive psychologic approaches, but more information about clinical effectiveness and whether any particular therapies have any specific advantages over other approaches is needed.

The basic aims of therapy in BP are to alleviate acute symptoms, restore psychosocial functioning, and prevent relapse and recurrence. The mainstay of treatment has been and currently remains pharmacotherapy. There is, however, a significant efficacy-effectiveness gap in the reported response rates to all mood stabilizers [1–5]; even under optimal clinical conditions, prophylaxis protects fewer than 50% of individuals with BP against further episodes [2,5–7]. Given this scenario, the development of specific psychologic therapies for BP seems to be a necessary and welcome advance. Until recently, however, progress in this area was slow.

Historically, individuals with BP were not offered psychologic therapies for three main reasons [7]. First, etiologic models highlighting genetic and

---

* Corresponding author. Division of Psychological Medicine, Institute of Psychiatry, P.O. Box 96, Denmark Hill, London 8E5 8AF, UK.
E-mail address: j.scott@iop.kcl.ac.uk (J. Scott).

biologic factors in BP have dominated the research agenda and largely dictated that medication was not merely the primary, but the only appropriate treatment. Second, there was a misconception that virtually all patients with BP made a full inter-episode recovery and returned to their premorbid level of functioning. Third, psychoanalysts historically expressed greater ambivalence about the suitability for psychotherapy of individuals with BP than those with other severe mental disorders. Fromm-Reichman [8] suggested that, in comparison with individuals with schizophrenia, patients with BP were poor candidates for psychotherapy because they lacked introspection, were too dependent, and were likely to discover and then play on the therapist's Achilles' heel. Others, particularly patients and their family members, argued strongly in favor of the use of psychologic treatments [2,9], but the relative lack of empiric support (before the last 5 years, few randomized, controlled trials had been published) meant that clinicians had few indicators of when or how to incorporate such approaches into day-to-day practice.

During the last decade, two key aspects have changed. First, there is increasing acceptance of stress-vulnerability models that highlight the interplay between psychologic, social, and biologic factors in the maintenance or frequency of recurrence of episodes of severe mental disorders. Second, evidence has accumulated from randomized, controlled treatment trials regarding the benefits of psychologic therapies as an adjunct to medication in treatment-resistant schizophrenia and in severe and chronic depressive disorders [10–12]. Although there has been only limited research on the use of similar interventions in BP, there are encouraging reports from research groups exploring the role of manualized therapies in this population [13]. For persons with BP who reported about 25 years ago that psychotherapy could help them adjust to the disorder and overcome barriers to the acceptance of pharmacotherapy [2], these developments are long overdue.

This article briefly outlines the rationale for using psychologic therapies in combination with standard approaches (usually outpatient support and medication) in the treatment of adult clients with BP. Outcome data from randomized, controlled trials are reviewed, and the characteristics of therapies that are efficacious in BP are highlighted. Finally, the authors comment on some of the issues involved in translating research efficacy into clinical effectiveness.

The rationale for adjunctive psychologic treatments

Recent studies of clinical populations of BP identify significant types of morbidity that may impair medication response rates or may simply be medication refractory [9]. Like persons with chronic medical disorders such as diabetes, hypertension, and epilepsy, 30% to 50% of individuals with BP do not adhere to prescribed prophylactic treatments. A greater proportion of the variance in adherence behavior is attributable to attitudes and beliefs about BP than to medication side effects or practical problems with the treatment regime [4,5]. Thirty percent to 50% of individuals with BP also meet criteria for substance misuse or personality disorders, which usually predict poorer response to medication alone. Many of these disorders precede the diagnosis of BP. BP has a median age of onset in the mid-20s, but most individuals report that they experienced symptoms or problems up to 10 years before diagnosis. Thus, the early evolution of BP may impair the process of normal personality development or may lead the person to employ maladaptive behaviors from adolescence onwards. The sleep patterns of persons with BP compared with healthy control subjects may indicate that such individuals have above-average sensitivity to circadian rhythm disruptions in response to social dysregulation [14–17]. Comorbid anxiety disorders (including panic and posttraumatic stress disorder) and other mental health problems are common accompaniments of BP, and 40% to 50% of patients may have inter-episode subsyndromal depression [18]. Individuals with BP also show abnormalities in cognitive style compared with healthy controls, with a more fluctuating and fragile self-esteem and above-average levels of perfectionism and desire for social approval and achievement [19]. Although many individuals manage to complete tertiary education and establish a career path, they may then experience loss of status or employment after repeated relapses. One year after an episode of BP, only 30% of individuals have returned to their previous level of social and vocational functioning. Interpersonal relationships may be damaged or lost because of behaviors during a manic episode, or the individual may struggle to overcome guilt or shame related to such acts.

Although this brief discussion highlights only some of the many problems associated with BP, it is helpful when considering the potential use of psychologic treatments. For example, psychoeducation can be used to enhance awareness of illness, to teach healthy living habits (reduce alcohol consumption, enhance medication adherence), and to reduce stigmatization [20,21]. A relapse-prevention package might be used to teach the individual to recognize the key early warning signs of BP relapse such as marked sleep disruption [22]. Interpersonal social rhythms therapy (IPSRT) can be used to stabilize circadian rhythms [16,17,23]. Cognitive therapy may be used to target self-esteem, reduce perfectionism, or enhance basic problem-solving skills [24–26]. These therapies do not map exclusively to one particular problem area; the boundaries between therapies are flexible, and there are several common elements. For example, cognitive therapy also addresses attitudes toward medication adherence and employs self-regulation techniques. IPSRT explores an individual's understanding of BP and beliefs about relationships or personal roles that may otherwise impair functioning. Family therapy may target a number of problems simultaneously, including malevolent interpretations and attributions made by other family members that may increase the risk of BP relapse in an at-risk individual [27,28].

Studies of psychologic treatments in bipolar disorders

Early treatment studies

There is a large literature of individual case studies and case series on the use of a variety of psychologic therapies in BP. Between 1960 and 1998, 32 outcome studies describing the combined use of psychologic and pharmacologic treatments in BP were published. Most, however, were small in scale, with an average sample size around 25. The total sample for all studies was just over 1000 participants, of whom about 75% received the experimental or novel psychologic treatment. Most of the reports addressed group (45%) or family (45%) approaches; only 15% reported on individual therapy. Less than half of all studies were randomized, controlled trials, and there were various other methodologic limitations. In many of these studies, however, it was clear that those receiving adjunctive psychologic treatments had better subjective and objective clinical and social outcomes than those receiving usual psychiatric care (consisting mainly of treatment with mood stabilizers and outpatient support), and that many of these differences reached statistical significance [7]. These encouraging results facilitated the development of randomized, controlled trials of more targeted interventions that primarily focused on the issue of BP relapse.

In the last 5 years, interest in psychosocial interventions in BP has increased dramatically with about 20 randomized, controlled trials underway in the United States, the United Kingdom, and Europe. Given the current emphasis on the use of brief, evidence-based therapies in clinical guidelines for the treatment of unipolar disorders, it is not surprising that the new treatment trials for BP have focused on psychoeducational models, on the three best-researched manualized psychologic approaches—IPSRT, cognitive therapy, and family focused therapy (FFT)—or on techniques derived directly from these therapies. Core studies from each of these approaches are reviewed here.

Key randomized, controlled treatment trials

Brief technique-driven interventions

There are two randomized, controlled trials of brief 6- to 12-session interventions delivered on an individual basis to persons with BP. Each study compared the experimental intervention with treatment as usual (usually medication plus outpatient support), and each study followed up participants for at least 12 months. Cochran [29] undertook a small trial that compared 28 patients who were randomly assigned to standard clinical care alone or to standard clinical care plus a six-session intervention that used cognitive and behavioral techniques to improve medication adherence. Following treatment, enhanced lithium adherence was reported in the intervention group, with only three patients (21%) discontinuing medication, as compared with eight patients (57%) in the group receiving standard clinical care alone. There were also fewer hospitalizations in the group receiving cognitive therapy (two versus eight). Unfortunately, no information was available on the nature of any affective relapses.

Perry and colleagues [22] recruited 69 participants at high risk of further relapse of BP who were in regular contact with mental health services in the United Kingdom. Individuals were randomly assigned to usual treatment or to usual treatment plus 6 to 12 sessions teaching cognitive and behavioral techniques that helped individuals identify and manage early warning signs of relapse. The problem-solving strategies included identification of high-risk situations and of prodromal symptoms (the relapse signature) and taught clients to self-medicate and to access mental health professionals at the earliest possible time to try to avert the development of full-blown episodes. Over 18 months, the results demonstrated that, in comparison to the control group, the intervention group had significantly fewer manic relapses (27% versus 57%), significantly fewer days in hospital, significantly longer time to first manic relapse (65 weeks versus 17 weeks), higher levels of social functioning, and better work performance.

Group psychoeducation

Van Gent and colleagues [30–32] undertook two randomized trials using a group-therapy format for individuals with BP and one trial of psycho-education for the partners of individuals with BP. The first study [30] allocated 20 participants with BP to four sessions of 90 minutes of group psychoeducation and 14 other participants to a waiting-list control condition (usual treatment). Each group was followed for 15 months. More individuals in the intervention group (75%) than the control group (29%) reported significant subjective improvements in self-confidence, and those receiving psychoeducation demonstrated significant improvements in behavior and social functioning. The groups were similar, however, in mood, anxiety, and general symptom ratings. In the second study, van Gent and Zwart [31] randomly assigned 15 participants to five sessions of psychoeducation and 20 other participants to 10 sessions of psycho-education plus psychotherapy. At 15-month follow-up, both groups showed improved psychosocial functioning, but the group that had received the extended intervention demonstrated a greater improvement in their thinking and behavior as measured on a general symptom checklist. The last study by van Gent and Zwart [32] explored the benefits of providing five structured group sessions for 14 partners of individuals with BP and compared their knowledge of BP, its treatment, and psychosocial management strategies over 6 months with 12 partners who were randomly allocated to a control condition. The study demonstrated that participants in the partner-only education sessions gained and sustained a significantly greater significant finding, however, was that the individuals with BP became significantly more anxious after the partner attended the experimental group without them. This understanding of BP than those allocated to the control group.

Perhaps the most finding suggests that individuals with BP may benefit from attending group psychoeducation sessions, but it may be more appropriate to use family sessions if the goal is for both partners and the individual with BP to benefit.

Colom et al [20,21] have undertaken the largest group therapy study so far. One hundred twenty participants with BP who were euthymic and receiving medication and standard outpatient follow-up were randomly assigned to either 20 sessions of group psychoeducation (approximately 8–12 individuals per group) or to an unstructured support group. Sessions were 90 minutes in duration and were conducted by two experienced clinical psychologists. Overall, when the mean number of relapses per subject, the total relapses per group, time to first relapse, length of hospitalization, and serum lithium levels were evaluated, there were clear and statistically significant advantages to psychoeducation as compared with the nondirective group. Reductions in depressive relapses were particularly noticeable and were significantly lower in both the treatment phase (psychoeducation 12% versus control 31%) and the follow-up phase (31% versus 71%, respectively). There was a similar significant reduction in relapse rates into hypomania and the same trend, which sometimes reached significance, for manic and mixed states. A recent subanalysis of the study data shows that psychoeducation may be useful even in those complex patients fulfilling criteria for a comorbid personality disorder [33].

Family or couples' therapy

Four small, randomized trials all indicated that family therapy may be an important adjunct to pharmacotherapy in BP. Honig and colleagues [34] demonstrated that six sessions of a multifamily psychoeducational intervention (n = 23) produced a nonsignificantly greater reduction in expressed emotion in the experimental group when compared with the waiting-list control group (n = 23). Van Gent et al [35] compared couples' psychoeducation (n = 14) with usual treatment (n = 12) and found that couples receiving the active intervention showed greater knowledge of BP and its treatment and improved coping skills at the end of the psychoeducation sessions and at 6-month follow-up. Glick et al [36] studied 50 inpatients, 19 of whom had been admitted following a BP relapse. They demonstrated that those randomly allocated to additional family therapy (n = 12) showed significant improvements in social and work functioning and in family attitudes compared with those who received usual inpatient care alone (n = 7). These gains were particularly noticeable in females with BP, and many of the immediate benefits associated with family therapy were maintained at 18-month follow-up [37]. Clarkin et al [38] randomly assigned 42 outpatients to 11 months of standard treatment (n = 23) or standard treatment plus 25 sessions of couples' therapy (n = 19). Unfortunately, the analysis was restricted to 33 treatment completers (couples' therapy, 18; control treatment, 15). Completing a course of couples' therapy was associated with significantly higher levels of social adjustment and medication adherence as compared with the control group, although there were no differences in overall symptom levels in the groups.

Miklowitz and colleagues [26,27] undertook the largest trial of family therapy using their 20-session FFT model. One hundred one participants with BP who were receiving usual treatment were randomly allocated to FFT (n = 31) or to case management (n = 70), which consisted of two sessions of family psychoeducation and crisis intervention as required. Over a 12-month period, individuals receiving FFT plus usual treatment survived significantly longer in the community without relapsing than those receiving case management plus usual treatment (71% versus 47%) and showed significantly greater reductions in symptom levels. Further analysis, however, demonstrated that these benefits were limited to depression, and there was no specific reduction in manic relapses or symptoms. Overall, the benefits of FFT were most striking in individuals living in an environment of high expressed emotion.

Interpersonal social rhythms therapy

The IPSRT intervention was one of the first systematic psychologic therapies developed specifically for individuals with BP. A randomized treatment trial with a 2-year follow-up is underway. Interim reports are available on 82 participants initially allocated to IPSRT or intensive clinical management. The trial has two phases: an acute-treatment phase and a maintenance phase. Fifty percent of the participants in each group remain in the same treatment arm throughout the study; the remaining participants cross over to the other treatment arm [23,39]. The key findings so far are that IPSRT does induce more stable social rhythms [16,17]. The differences between treatments in time to remission were not statistically significant, but those in the IPSRT group who entered the trial during a major depressive episode showed a significantly shorter time to recovery than those in the intensive clinical management group (21 weeks versus 40 weeks). Patients receiving the same treatment throughout the acute and maintenance phases of the study showed greater reductions in symptoms, suicide attempts, and total number of relapses than those who were assigned to the crossover condition. This finding suggests that consistency in treatment is more important than type of treatment alone.

Cognitive therapy

A study by Scott et al [24] examined the effect of 20 sessions of cognitive therapy in 42 clients with BP. Participants could enter the study during any phase of BP. Clients were initially randomly allocated to the intervention group or to a waiting-list control group who received cognitive therapy after a 6-month delay. The randomized phase (6 months) allowed assessment of the effects of cognitive therapy plus usual treatment as compared with usual treatment alone. Individuals from both groups were monitored for a further

12 months after cognitive therapy. At initial assessment, 30% of participants met criteria for an affective episode: 11 participants met diagnostic criteria for depressive disorder, 3 for rapid cycling disorder, 3 for hypomania, and 1 for a mixed state. As is typical of this client population, 12 participants also met criteria for drug or alcohol problems or dependence, 2 met criteria for other Axis I disorders, and about 60% of the sample met criteria for personality disorder. The results of the randomized, controlled phase demonstrated that, compared with participants receiving treatment as usual, those who received additional cognitive therapy experienced statistically significant improvements in symptom levels, global functioning, and work and social adjustment. Data were available from 29 participants who received cognitive therapy and were followed for 12 months after cognitive therapy. These patients demonstrated a 60% reduction in relapse rates in the 18 months after commencing cognitive therapy as compared with the 18 months before receiving cognitive therapy. Hospitalization rates showed parallel reductions. Scott et al concluded that cognitive therapy plus treatment as usual may offer some benefit and is a highly acceptable treatment intervention to about 70% of clients with BP. This study was the forerunner of a large five-center trial of treatment as usual versus cognitive therapy plus treatment as usual. The sample (n = 250) is the largest for a psychologic therapy in BP. Results will be available in the near future.

Lam and colleagues [25] followed up their pilot study (25 participants randomly assigned to cognitive therapy or to usual treatment) of 12 to 20 sessions of outpatient cognitive therapy for BP with a large-scale, randomized, controlled trial [26]. One hundred three participants with BP who were currently euthymic were randomly allocated to individual cognitive therapy as an adjunct to mood-stabilizing medication or to usual treatment alone (mood stabilizers plus outpatient support). After controlling for gender and illness history, the intervention group had significantly fewer BP relapses (cognitive therapy group 43%; control group 75%), psychiatric admissions (15% versus 33%) or total days in episode (about 27 days versus 88 days) over 12 months than the control group. The reduction in total number of episodes comprised significant reductions in major depressive (21% versus 52%) and manic (17% versus 31%) episodes but not in mixed episodes. The intervention group also showed significantly greater improvements in social adjustment and better coping strategies for managing prodromal symptoms of mania.

Overview of therapy outcome trials: similarities and differences

As shown in Table 1, the use of adjunctive therapy leads to significant reductions in relapse rates and symptom levels and significant improvements in social functioning. Scott and Gutierrez [40] pooled the data from eight of the studies reviewed to undertake a meta-analysis of the impact of adjunctive therapy on relapse rates for the 12 months after entry into the

Table 1
Key randomized, controlled trials of the five main models of psychologic therapies of bipolar disorders

Study	Sample size	Experimental intervention	Main differences in outcome between experimental and control treatments
Perry et al, 1999	69	Relapse prevention using cognitive and behavioral strategies	Reduced lengths of hospitalization. Increased time between episodes. More effective in preventing relapses into mania. No effect on depression
Frank et al, 1999	82	Interpersonal social rhythms therapy (IPSRT)	Increased stability of social rhythms. More effect on depression, with trend towards shorter time to recovery from a major depressive episode. No effect on manic relapse.
Miklowitz et al, 2003	101	Family focused therapy (FFT)	Significantly fewer relapses but more effective in reducing depression than mania. FFT particularly helpful in families with high levels of expressed emotion.
Lam et al, 2003	103	Cognitive therapy	Significantly fewer episodes of mania and depression. Improved social functioning. Greater awareness and better coping with manic prodromes
Colom et al, 2003	120	Group psychoeducation	Significantly fewer BP episodes (manic, depressive, and mixed). Greatest effect on depression, but also hypomania

treatment trial compared with relapse rates in individuals allocated to standard treatment alone (outpatient follow-up plus medication). The findings from the IPSRT cross-over trial should be treated with caution, given the different design and the enhanced standard treatment received in this study. That study aside, Fig. 1 shows that the benefits of each psychologic treatment are largely comparable and that there is a highly significant reduction in relapses when these therapies are provided in addition to standard treatments (random effects model: odds ratio, 0.38; 95% confidence interval, 0.22–0.66; $P = 0.001$).

This review demonstrates that therapies sometimes differed in their relative effectiveness in reducing depressive or manic relapses. The reasons are not entirely clear, but at least two hypotheses can be suggested. First, there may be different active ingredients in the therapies that more successfully tackle the syndrome of depression or mania. Alternatively, as Jackson et al [41] noted, the symptoms of manic relapse are qualitatively different from day-to-day experiences, whereas depressive prodromes often

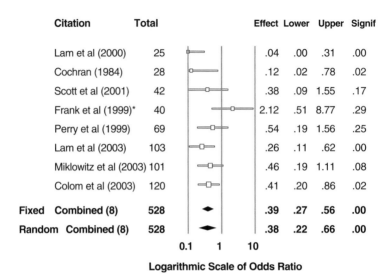

Citation	Total		Effect	Lower	Upper	Signif
Lam et al (2000)	25		.04	.00	.31	.00
Cochran (1984)	28		.12	.02	.78	.02
Scott et al (2001)	42		.38	.09	1.55	.17
Frank et al (1999)*	40		2.12	.51	8.77	.29
Perry et al (1999)	69		.54	.19	1.56	.25
Lam et al (2003)	103		.26	.11	.62	.00
Miklowitz et al (2003)	101		.46	.19	1.11	.08
Colom et al (2003)	120		.41	.20	.86	.02
Fixed Combined (8)	528		.39	.27	.56	.00
Random Combined (8)	528		.38	.22	.66	.00

0.1   1   10

Logarithmic Scale of Odds Ratio

Fig. 1. Meta-analysis of published trials psychological therapy plus outpatient follow-up and medication compared to outpatient follow-up and medication alone. * The 40 subjects in the meta-analysis represent the subgroup of trial participants who remained either in the IPSRT or in the intensive clinical management arm throughout the study period.

represent quantitative variations from normal experience. Mania also has a longer prodrome than depression (median time, approximately 3 weeks as compared with 2 weeks). Interventions that focus primarily on teaching individuals to recognize early warning symptoms and to make effective interventions (eg, behavior change or increases in medication) may prevent isolated manic symptoms from cascading into a full-blown maniac relapse but may be less effective in identifying a depressive prodrome and intervening in a timely manner [41]. Interventions that tackle subsyndromal or acute BP depression often require complex, multifaceted approaches such as those included in cognitive behavior therapy and interpersonal psychotherapy and already known to be effective in the treatment of unipolar depression.

Although the randomized trials reviewed here are relatively small in comparison to medication trials, there is encouraging evidence for the clinical efficacy of each key approach. In addition, randomized trials of group therapies targeting comorbid BP and substance misuse [42] or using Bauer and colleagues' [43] life goals program are nearing completion and will further enhance the understanding of which approach works for whom.

Summary

Psychosocial problems may be causes or consequences of BP relapses, and adding psychologic therapies to usual-treatment approaches may improve the prognosis of those at risk of persistent symptoms or frequent episodes. The three core individual manualized therapies (IPSRT, cognitive therapy, and FFT) have all developed specific models for use in BP. Colom et al's [21] group psychoeducation model also has a clearly developed rationale and format, and it allows individuals to share their views of BP with others, to learn adaptive coping strategies from the other 8 to 12 members of the group, and to have regular contact with an expert therapist.

Careful review of the four more extended and comprehensive approaches and the brief technique-driven interventions demonstrates that the effective therapies incorporate one or more of the modules show in Box 1. At present, the choice between the four extended models is more likely to be dictated by patient choice or the availability of a trained therapist. The technique-driven interventions are briefer than the specific therapies (about 6–9 sessions compared with about 20–22 sessions) and usually offer a generic, fixed treatment package targeted at a circumscribed issue such as medication adherence or managing early symptoms of relapse. These brief interventions can be delivered by a less-skilled or less-experienced professional than the specific model. They potentially seem to be useful in day-to-day clinical practice in general adult psychiatry settings; additional larger-scale, randomized trials should be encouraged.

Given the reduction in relapse rates and hospitalizations associated with the use of psychologic therapy as an adjunct to medication, it is likely that these approaches will prove to be clinically and cost effective. They may provide a significant improvement in the quality of life of individuals with BP (and indirectly to that of their partners and family members). Brief, evidence-based therapies represent an important component of good clinical practice in the management of BP. Studies of a comprehensive, whole-system approach to the collaborative psychobiosocial management of BP are being undertaken in the United States [43]. If these approaches improve the quality and continuity of care for individuals with BP, they will have further implications for the delivery and organization of mental health services.

The number and variety of trials of psychosocial interventions is exciting for researchers and clinicians interested in BP. Enthusiasm for advocating these approaches should be tempered by an acknowledgment that the trials undertaken so far largely demonstrate efficacy in selected samples of patients treated at specialist BP clinics or psychologic treatment research

---

Box 1. Shared targets for psychologic treatments

1. Psychoeducation about the disorder
2. Lifestyle regularity (including reduction in substance use)
3. Adherence to medication regimen
4. Early recognition and management of symptoms of relapse

centers. Translating efficacy into effectiveness requires evidence that the approaches used in the treatment trials are equally beneficial when used by the wider therapist community treating patients seen routinely in non-specialist or nonresearch centers. These patients often have multiple problems or complex presentations that preclude their involvement in pharmacologic or psychologic treatment studies, but monitoring the outcomes of these representative samples will be important in determining the true place of psychologic approaches in the management of BP [44]. Large-scale studies are now underway on both sides of the Atlantic (the Medical Research Council study in the United Kingdom and the STEP-BD project in the United States). These trials are likely to answer basic questions about the benefits and limitations of psychologic therapies in the acute and maintenance treatment of BP in the clinical realm and will increase understanding of the effectiveness-versus-efficacy question.

References

[1] Guscott R, Taylor L. Lithium prophylaxis in recurrent affective illness: efficacy, effectiveness and efficiency. Br J Psychiatry 1994;164:741–6.
[2] Jamison KR, Garner RH, Goodwin FK. Patient and physician attitudes toward lithium. Arch Gen Psychiatry 1979;36:866–9.
[3] Scott J. Cognitive therapy for depression. Br Med Bull 2001;57:101–13.
[4] Scott J, Pope M. Non-adherence with mood-stabilizers: prevalence and predictors. J Clin Psychiatry 2002;65:384–90.
[5] Colom F, Vieta E, Martínez-Arán A, et al. Clinical factors associated to treatment non-compliance in euthymic bipolar patients. J Clin Psychiatry 2000;61:549–54.
[6] Dickson WE, Kendell RE. Does maintenance lithium therapy prevent recurrences of mania under ordinary clinical conditions? Psychol Med 1994;16:521–30.
[7] Scott J. Psychotherapy for bipolar disorder: an unmet need? Br J Psychiatry 1995;167:581–8.
[8] Fromm-Reichman F. Intensive psychotherapy of manic-depressives: a preliminary report. Confina Neurologica 1949;9:158–65.
[9] Goodwin F, Jamison K. Manic depressive illness. Oxford (UK): Oxford University Press; 1990. p. 530–2.
[10] Paykel E, Scott J, Teasdale J, et al. Prevention of relapse in residual depression by cognitive therapy: a controlled trial. Arch Gen Psychiatry 1999;56:829–35.
[11] Sensky T, Turkington D, Kingdon D, et al. A randomised controlled trial of cognitive behavioural therapy for persistent symptoms in schizophrenia resistant to medication. Arch Gen Psychiatry 2000;57:165–72.
[12] Thase ME, Greenhouse JB, Frank E. Treatment of major depression with psychotherapy or psychotherapy-pharmacotherapy combinations. Arch Gen Psychiatry 1997;54:1009–15.
[13] American Psychiatric Association. Practice guideline for the treatment of patients with bipolar disorders. Am J Psychiatry 1994;151(Suppl);1–36.
[14] Miller A, Espie C, Scott J. Actigraphy of sleep patterns in individuals with bipolar disorders compared to healthy controls. J Affect Disord, in press.
[15] Ehlers C, Frank E, Kupfer D. Social zeitgebers and biological rhythms: a unified approach to understanding the etiology of depression. Arch Gen Psychiatry 1988;45:948–52.

[16] Frank E, Swartz HA, Kupfer DJ. Interpersonal and social rhythm therapy: managing the chaos of bipolar disorder. Biol Psychiatry 2000;48:593–604.

[17] Frank E, Hlastala S, Ritenour A, et al. Inducing lifestyle regularity in recovering bipolar patients: results from the maintenance therapies in bipolar disorder protocol. Biol Psychiatry 1994;41:1165–73.

[18] Judd LL, Akiskal HS, Schlettler PJ, et al. The long-term natural history of the weekly symptomatic status of bipolar I disorder. Arch Gen Psychiatry 2002;59:530–7.

[19] Scott J. Cognitive therapy as an adjunct to medication in bipolar disorders. Br J Psychiatry (Suppl) 2001;178:S164–8.

[20] Colom F, Martinez-Aran A, Reinares M, et al. Psychoeducation and prevention of relapse in bipolar disorders: preliminary results. Bipolar Disord 2001;3(Suppl):32.

[21] Colom F, Vieta E, Martinez-Aran A, et al. A randomized trial of group psychoeducation in bipolar disorder. Arch Gen Psychiatry 2003;60:402–7.

[22] Perry A, Tarrier N, Morriss R, et al. Randomized controlled trial of efficacy of teaching patients with bipolar disorder to identify early symptoms of relapse and obtain treatment. BMJ 1999;318:149–53.

[23] Frank E, Swartz H, Mallinger A, et al. Adjunctive psychotherapy for bipolar disorder: effect of changing treatment modality. J Abnorm Psychol 1999;108:579–87.

[24] Scott J, Garland A, Moorhead S. A pilot study of cognitive therapy in bipolar disorder. Psychol Med 2001;31:459–67.

[25] Lam D, Bright J, Jones S, et al. Cognitive therapy for bipolar illness—a pilot study of relapse prevention. Cognit Ther Res 2000;24:503–20.

[26] Lam D, Bright J, Jones S, et al. A randomized controlled trial of cognitive therapy for relapse prevention in bipolar disorders. Arch Gen Psychiatry 2003;60:145–52.

[27] Miklowitz D, Simoneau T, George E, et al. Family focused treatment of bipolar disorder: 1-year effects of a psychoeducational program in conjunction with pharmacotherapy. Biol Psychiatry 2000;48:582–92.

[28] Miklowitz DJ, George EL, Richards JA, et al. A randomized study of family-focused psychoeducation and pharmacotherapy in the outpatient management of bipolar disorder. Arch Gen Psychiatry 2003;60:904–12.

[29] Cochran S. Preventing medication non-compliance in the outpatient treatment of bipolar affective disorders. J Consult Clin Psychol 1984;52:873–8.

[30] Van Gent E, Vida S, Zwart F. Group therapy in addition to lithium in patients with bipolar disorders. Acta Psychiatr Belg 1988;88:405–18.

[31] Van Gent E, Zwart F. Psychoeducation of partners of bipolar manic patients. J Affect Disord 1991;21:15–8.

[32] Van Gent E, Zwart F. Ultra-short versus short group therapy in addition to lithium. Patient Educ Couns 1993;21:135–41.

[33] Colom F, Vieta E, Sánchez-Moreno J, et al. Psychoeducation in bipolar patients with comorbid personality disorders. Bipolar Disord 2004;6:294–8.

[34] Honig A, Hofman A, Rozendaal N, et al. Psychoeducation in bipolar disorder: effect on expressed emotion. Psychiatry Res 1997;72:17–22.

[35] Van Gent E, Vogtlander L, Vrendendaal J. Two group psychoeducation programs compared. Toronto: American Psychiatric Association; 1998.

[36] Glick I, Burti L, Okonogi K, et al. Effectiveness in psychiatric care: psychoeducation and outcome for patients with major affective disorder and their families. Br J Psychiatry 1994; 164:104–6.

[37] Haas G, Glick I, Clarkin J. Inpatient family intervention: a randomized clinical trial. Results at hospital discharge. Arch Gen Psychiatry 1988;45:217–24.

[38] Clarkin J, Carpenter D, Hull J, et al. Effects of psychoeducation for married patients with bipolar disorder and their spouses. Psychiatr Serv 1998;49:531–3.

[39] Hlastata S, Frank E, Mallinger A, et al. Bipolar depression: an underestimated treatment challenge. Depress Anxiety 1997;5:73–83.

[40] Scott J, Guitierrez M. A systematic review of the benefits of current psychological therapies in bipolar disorders. Bipolar Disord, in press.

[41] Jackson A, Cavanagh J, Scott J. A systematic review of prodromal symptoms of mania and depression. J Affect Disord 2003;74:209–17.

[42] Weiss R, Kolodziej M, Najavits L, et al. Utilization of psychosocial treatments by patients diagnosed with bipolar disorder and substance misuse. Am J Addict 2000;9:314–20.

[43] Bauer M, McBride L, Chase C, et al. Manual-based group psychotherapy for bipolar disorder: a feasibility study. J Clin Psychiatry 1997;59:439–45.

[44] Scott J. Psychological therapies in bipolar disorders: does the evidence stack up? Journal of Neuropsychopharmacology, in press.

ELSEVIER
SAUNDERS

Psychiatr Clin N Am
28 (2005) 385–397

PSYCHIATRIC
CLINICS
OF NORTH AMERICA

Pharmacotherapy of Children and Adolescents with Bipolar Disorder

Robert A. Kowatch, MD[a,b,*], Melissa P. DelBello, MD[a,b]

[a]Cincinnati Children's Hospital Medical Center, Cincinnati, OH, USA
[b]Department of Psychiatry, University of Cincinnati Medical Center, Cincinnati, OH, USA

Pediatric bipolar disorder is a serious disorder that seriously disrupts the lives of children and adolescents [1,2]. Children and adolescents with a bipolar disorder have significantly higher rates of morbidity and mortality, including psychosocial morbidity with impaired family and peer relationships [3], impaired academic performance with increased rates of school failure and school dropout [4], increased levels of substance abuse, increased rates of suicide attempts and completion, legal difficulties, and multiple hospitalizations [2,5]. Children and adolescents with a bipolar disorder are often brought to clinical attention because of their severe mood swings, disruptive behaviors, short sleep periods, intrusiveness, and hypersexuality. These disorders generally present differently than adult bipolar disorders because of developmental differences in the expression of this disorder in children and adolescents.

In a study of the incidence of mood disorders in adolescents in six Oregon high schools, Lewinsohn et al [1] reported an overall lifetime prevalence of 1% for bipolar disorders, which included bipolar I disorder, bipolar II disorder, and cyclothymia. In this study, the largest groups of adolescent subjects were what Lewinsohn and colleagues [1] called the core-positive group. These adolescents reported a distinct period of elevated, expansive, or irritable mood and best fit the *Diagnostic and Statistical Manual-IV* (DSM-IV) criteria for bipolar disorder, not otherwise specified (NOS). These subjects had an overall prevalence of 5.7% and accounted for 84% of Lewinsohn's bipolar sample [1]. Like the bipolar I subjects, the bipolar NOS subjects had high rates of psychosocial impairment and mental health service use. In more specialized

---

* Corresponding author. Department of Psychiatry, University of Cincinnati Medical Center, MSB 7261, P.O. Box 670559, Cincinnati, OH 45267.
E-mail address: Robert.Kowatch@uc.edu (R.A. Kowatch).

psychiatric settings, such as a pediatric psychopharmacology clinic, the occurrence of bipolar disorder is often much greater than that found in the general population. Wozniak et al [6] reported that of 16% of 262 consecutively referred children to a specialty pediatric psychopharmacology clinic met DSM-III-R criteria for mania. Isaac et al [7] reported that 8 of 12 students in a special education class met DSM-IIIR criteria for a bipolar disorder. In child/adolescent psychiatric inpatient units, it is common to find 30% to 40% of patients with a bipolar disorder.

Diagnosis of pediatric bipolar disorders

Children with bipolar disorder often present with a mixed or dysphoric picture characterized by frequent short periods of intense mood lability and irritability rather than classic euphoric mania [6,8]. Geller and colleagues [9] recently reported the results of a 4-year prospective study of 86 prepubescent and early-adolescent subjects. These subjects were evaluated every 4 months across a 4-year period by a research nurse using the Washington University Kiddie Schedule for Affective Disorders and Schizophrenia (WASH-U-K-SADS) [10]. To differentiate mania from attention deficit hyperactivity disorder (ADHD) clearly, Geller et al required the presence of elated mood or grandiosity in bipolar subjects. They defined an episode of mania as the entire length of the illness, with cycles of manic symptoms as short as 4 hours and with at least one cycle daily for 2 weeks, meeting DSM-IV criteria for mania. In this well-characterized sample, 10% had ultrarapid cycling, and 77% had ultradian (daily) mood cycling. None of these cases met DSM-IV criteria for rapid cycling (four or more episodes per year) but were described as having 3.5 ± 2.0 cycles (mood swings) per day. The average age of onset for mania/hypomania was 7.4 ± 3.5 years, with an average episode length of 79.2 ± 66.7 weeks. This study revealed that, in this sample of children and adolescents with more classic mania with euphoria and grandiosity, the phenomenology of mania is different from that seen in adults.

Bipolar II disorder with clearly defined episodes of hypomania and depression presents more often in adolescents than in children, who usually present with a major depressive episode. Past episodes of hypomania may be missed unless a careful history is taken. Cyclothymia is difficult to diagnose, because the hypomania and depressive symptoms are not as severe as in bipolar I or bipolar II disorder. Prospective mood charting is often helpful to diagnose cyclothymia. Bipolar NOS represents the largest group of patients with bipolar symptoms, and this diagnosis is made when the patient's bipolar symptoms are present but are not of sufficient severity or duration to warrant a diagnosis of bipolar I, II, or cyclothymia. Alternately, the diagnosis of bipolar NOS can be made when that a bipolar disorder is present but is secondary to a general medical condition (ie, fetal alcohol syndrome or alcohol-related neurodevelopmental disorder). A number of medications and medical disorders may exacerbate or mimic bipolar symptoms, and it is important to assess these potential confounders before initiating treatment. Potential medical disorders and medications that should be evaluated before making the diagnosis of a bipolar disorder in children and adolescents are listed in Box 1.

Comorbid disorders

Comorbid disorders are the rule rather than the exception among children and adolescents with bipolar disorder. These comorbid disorders often complicate the presentation and treatment response. The most common comorbid diagnosis among children and adolescents with bipolar disorder is ADHD. Several studies have determined that ADHD is more common in prepubertal-onset bipolar disorder than in adolescent-onset bipolar disorder [11,12]. The rate of comorbid ADHD in prepubertal children is about 60% to 90%, whereas in adolescents the rate is 30% to 40%. Children with ADHD do not demonstrate the elated mood, grandiosity, hypersexuality, decreased need for sleep, racing thoughts, and other manic symptoms that are present in children with mania and comorbid ADHD [13].

Another common comorbid disorder in children with bipolar disorder is conduct disorder. Kovacs and Pollock [14] found a 69% rate of conduct

---

Box 1. Cofounders that may mimic mania in children and adolescents

Medical conditions that may mimic mania in children and adolescents
Temporal lobe epilepsy
Hyperthyroidism
Closed or open head injury
Multiple Sclerosis
Systemic lupus erythematosus
Wilson's disease

Medications that may increase mood cycling in children and adolescents
Antidepressants
• Tricyclic antidepressants
• Serotonin-specific reuptake inhibitors
• Serotonin and norepinephrine reuptake inhibitors
Aminophylline
Oral or intravenous corticosteroids
Sympathomimetic amines (eg, pseudoephedrine)
Antibiotics (eg, clarithromycin, erythromycin, and amoxicillin)

disorder among 26 bipolar children and adolescents. Moreover, adolescents with bipolar disorder are four to five times more likely to develop a substance use disorder than those without bipolar disorder [15]. Children and adolescents with pervasive developmental disorders may be at increased risk for developing mania [16].

Pharmacotherapy of bipolar disorders

The clinical use of traditional mood stabilizers and atypical antipsychotic agents in children and adolescents with bipolar disorders has increased significantly during the past few years, even though there are few controlled trials in this population. To date, there have been only two double-blind, placebo-controlled studies of the treatment for acute mania in children and adolescents with bipolar disorder [17,18] and one uncontrolled maintenance treatment study [19]. Nonetheless, many of the psychotropic medications used to treat adults with bipolar disorders also are used for children and adolescents with good responses. Information on dosing and clinical monitoring of the traditional and novel mood stabilizers is provided in Table 1.

Traditional mood stabilizers

Lithium

Lithium is the best-studied mood stabilizer for children and adolescents with bipolar disorder and is the only medication approved by the United States Food and Drug Administration for the treatment of acute mania and bipolar disorder in adolescents or children (ages 12–18 years). In the only prospective, placebo-controlled investigation of lithium in children and adolescents with bipolar disorders (N = 25), Geller et al [17] found that after 6 weeks of treatment, subjects treated with lithium showed a statistically significant decrease in positive urine toxicology screens and a significant improvement in global assessment of functioning (46% in the lithium-treated group versus 8% in the placebo group). This study demonstrated the efficacy of lithium carbonate for the treatment of bipolar adolescents with comorbid substance use disorders but did not measure the effect of lithium on mood in these adolescents. Clinical factors that predict a poor lithium response in children and adolescents with bipolar disorder include prepubertal onset and the presence of co-occurring ADHD [20]. Approximately 40% to 50% of children and adolescents with bipolar disorder respond acutely to lithium monotherapy [21–23]. In general, lithium should be titrated to a dose of 30 mg/kg/day in two to three divided doses, which typically results in a therapeutic serum level of 0.8 to 1.2 mEq/L. Common side effects of lithium in children and adolescents include hypothyroidism, nausea, polyuria, polydipsia, tremor, acne, and weight

Table 1
Mood stabilizer dosing/monitoring in children and adolescents with bipolar disorder

Generic name	United States trade name	How supplied (mg)	Starting dose	Target dose	Therapeutic serum level	Cautions
Carbamazepine Carbamazepine XR	Tegretol Tegretol XR	100, 200 100, 200, 400	Outpatients: 7 mg/kg/day 2–3 daily doses	Based on response and serum levels	8–11 mg/L	Watch for P450 drug interactions
Gabapentin	Neurontin	100, 300, 400	100 mg 2 ×/day or 3 ×/day	Based on response	NA	Watch for behavioral disinhibition
Lamotrigine	Lamictal	25, 100, 200	12.5 mg/day	Increase weekly based on response	NA	Monitor carefully for rashes, serum sickness
Lithium plus carbonate	Lithobid	300 (& 150 generic)	Outpatients: 25 mg/kg/day 2–3 daily doses	30 mg/kg/day 2–3 daily doses	0.8–1.2 mEq/L	Monitor for hypothyroidism avoid in pregnancy
Lithium plus carbonate	Eskalith	300 or 450 CR				
Lithium plus citrate	Cibaltih-S citrate	Lithium citrate 5 cm³ = 300 mg				
Oxcarbazepine	Trileptal	150, 300, 600	150 mg 2 ×/day	20–29 kg 900 mg/day 30–39 kg 1200 mg/day > 39 kg 1800 mg/day	NA	Monitor for hyponatremia
Topiramate	Topamax	25, 100	25 mg/day	100–400 mg/day	NA	Monitor for memory problems, kidney stones
Valproic acid Divalproex sodium	Depakene Depakote	125, 250, 500	20 mg/kg/day 2 daily doses	20 mg/kg/day 2–3 daily doses	90–120 mg/L	Monitor liver functions and for pancreatitis. avoid in pregnancy

Abbreviation: NA, not applicable.

gain. Lithium levels and renal and thyroid function should be monitored at baseline and every 6 months, as in adults.

Sodium divalproex

Despite the wide use of sodium divalproex in bipolar children and adolescents, there are no published placebo-controlled studies of divalproex in this population. Open-label studies of divalproex in manic adolescents have reported response rates ranging from 53% to 82% [21,24–26]. In bipolar children and adolescents, sodium divalproex can be initiated at a dose of 20 mg/kg/day, which typically produces a serum level of 80 to 120 µg/mL. Common side effects of divalproex in children are weight gain, nausea, sedation, and tremor. There has been much debate regarding the possible association between divalproex and polycystic ovarian syndrome (PCOS). The initial reports of PCOS were in women with epilepsy who were treated with divalproex [27]. The proposed mechanism for divalproex-induced PCOS is that obesity secondary to divalproex results in elevated insulin levels, which leads to increased androgen levels and ultimately to PCOS. Further investigations of the risk of developing PCOS for female bipolar adolescents are necessary. Until this issue is settled, clinicians should monitor female patients treated with divalproex for any signs of PCOS that include weight or menstrual abnormalities, hirsutism, or acne.

Carbamazepine

Carbamazepine has been used for seizure management in children and adolescents. Several case reports and series have described the successful use of carbamazepine as monotherapy and as adjunctive treatment in children and adolescents with bipolar disorder [28,29]. Carbamazepine must be titrated slowly and requires frequent monitoring of blood levels because of CYP450–drug interactions. Side effects of carbamazepine include aplastic anemia and severe dermatologic reactions such as Stevens-Johnson's syndrome, hyponatremia, nausea, and sedation. Carbamazepine therefore is less commonly used to treat children and adolescents with bipolar disorder [30]. Carbamazepine is usually titrated to a dose of 15 mg/kg/day to produce a serum level of 7 to 10 µg/mL. It is difficult to use carbamazepine with sodium divalproex because the CYP450–drug interaction with these two agents.

Novel antiepileptic agents

Several new antiepileptic agents developed for the treatment of epilepsy may have mood-stabilizing properties, but the data regarding the efficacy and tolerability of these agents for the treatment of pediatric bipolar disorder are limited at present. These novel antiepileptic drugs may be useful as adjuncts for the treatment of manic and hypomanic episodes. Oxcarbazepine, an analogue of carbamazepine, is a promising agent for treating acute mania in adults [31,32], but no pediatric data with this agent are available. There have been several reports of lamotrigine used as adjunctive treatment for children and adolescents with bipolar disorder [33], but this use has been limited because of the risk of potentially lethal cutaneous reactions such as Stevens-Johnson syndrome and toxic epidermal necrolysis. The risk of developing a serious rash is approximately two to three times greater in children and adolescents younger than 16 years old than in adults. A recent, more conservative dosing schedule seems to reduce the rate of serious rashes substantially, however [34,35]. Double-blind, placebo-controlled studies of gabapentin have demonstrated that gabapentin is no more effective than placebo for the treatment of acute mania in adults [36]. Gabapentin may be effective for the treatment of anxiety disorders in adults [37,38], however, and is generally well tolerated in children and adolescents. Gabapentin may be useful for treating children and adolescents with bipolar disorder who are also diagnosed with a comorbid anxiety disorder, but controlled data are lacking. Preliminary data from open studies suggest that topiramate [39] may be effective as an adjunctive treatment for pediatric bipolar disorder [40], although more recent double-blind, placebo-controlled studies in adults with mania suggest that as monotherapy it is no more effective than placebo. Word-finding difficulties have been reported in up to one third of patients treated with topiramate [41]. Topiramate is associated with anorexia and weight loss [42] and therefore may be useful as adjunctive treatment for children and adolescents with bipolar disorder who have gained weight as a result of treatment with other psychotropic medications.

Atypical antipsychotic agents

The atypical antipsychotic agents are powerful psychotropic drugs that have recently been found to be efficacious in the treatment of adults with schizophrenia, acute bipolar mania, bipolar depression, treatment-resistant depression, and posttraumatic stress disorder [43,44]. These atypical agents have antipsychotic activity and demonstrate mood-stabilizing properties with favorable effects on the depressive and manic symptoms of patients with bipolar disorders [45]. To date, there have been three large controlled studies of olanzapine [46–48], two controlled trials of risperidone [49,50], one controlled trial of aripiprazole [51], and one controlled trial of ziprasidone [52,53] in the treatment of adults with acute mania.

Several recent case series and open-label reports suggest that the atypical antipsychotic agents clozapine [54], risperidone [55], olanzapine [56–58], and quetiapine [18] are effective in the treatment of pediatric mania. Clinically, these agents seem more efficacious than the traditional mood stabilizers in children and adolescents with bipolar disorder. Currently, there are ongoing controlled trials of several atypical antipsychotic agents, including risperidone, olanzapine, and quetiapine, for the treatment of mania in children and adolescents. Information on dosing and clinical monitoring of atypical antipsychotic agents is provided in Table 2.

Table 2
Atypical antipsychotic agent dosing/monitoring in children and adolescents with bipolar
disorder

Generic name	United States trade name	How supplied (mg)	Pediatric starting dose (mg)	Target dose (mg/day)	Cautions
Clozapine	Clozaril	25, 100	25 2 ×/day	200–400	Monitor white blood cell count weekly; seizures possible at higher doses
Olanzapine	Zyprexa	2.5, 5, 7.5, 10, 15, 20	2.5 2 ×/day	10–20	Monitor weight, cholesterol
	Zydis	5			
Quetiapine	Seroquel	25, 100, 200	50 2 ×/day	400–600	
Risperidone	Risperdal	0.25, 0.5, 1, 2, 3, 4	0.25 2 ×/day	1–2	Monitor for extrapyramidal symptoms and galactorrhea
Ziprasidone	Geodon	20, 40, 60, 80	20 2 ×/day	80–120	Check baseline EKG and as dose increases
Aripiprazole	Abilify	2.5, 5, 10, 15, 25	2.5–5 at bedtime	10–25	Monitor for PY450 interactions (CYP3A4 & CYP2D6)

Despite their effectiveness, atypical antipsychotic agents are associated
with side effects. Like many agents used to treat children and adolescents
with bipolar disorder, clozapine and olanzapine frequently cause significant
weight gain in children and adolescents [59]. A series of general medical and
metabolic problems, including type II (non–insulin-dependent) diabetes
mellitus, changes in lipid levels, and transaminase elevation, may occur as
a result of weight gain [60,61]. Children who experience significant weight
gain should be monitored especially closely for these possibilities and should
be referred for exercise and nutritional counseling. Recently the American
Diabetes Association in collaboration with the American Psychiatric
Association published a monitoring protocol for all patients before initiating treatment with an atypical antipsychotic agent [62]. This protocol
includes obtaining a personal and family history of obesity, diabetes,
dyslipidemia, hypertension, or cardiovascular disease; weight and height so
that body mass index can be calculated; measurement of waist circumfer-
ence (at the level of the umbilicus); blood pressure; fasting plasma glucose;
and a fasting lipid profile. This group recommended that the patient's
weight should be reassessed at 4, 8, and 12 weeks after initiating or changing
therapy with an atypical antipsychotic agent and every 3 months thereafter

at the time of routine visits. If a patient gains more than 5% of his or her initial weight at any time during therapy, an alternative agent should be substituted. These guidelines should be followed in all children and adolescents treated with atypical antipsychotic agents. Although these guidelines are extremely helpful, they were not written for a pediatric population, and the 5% weight gain threshold may not be sensitive enough for children and adolescents. Ziprasidone [63] can cause QTc prolongation in children and adolescents [64]. Therefore, ziprasidone should be used with caution in children and adolescents with bipolar disorder, and EKGs should be monitored at baseline and when significant dosage increases are made.

Treatment strategies

The overall strategy when treating children and adolescents with bipolar disorder is to stabilize the mood and then treat other comorbid disorders such as ADHD. The majority of prepubertal children with a bipolar disorder present with mixed mania or hypomania that responds best to a traditional mood stabilizer such as valproate or an atypical antipsychotic agent. The atypical antipsychotic agents, because of their effectiveness and ease of use, are quickly becoming first-line treatments for mania and hypomania in children and adolescents. If a child or adolescent presents with a classic euphoric mania without psychotic symptoms, a trial of lithium may be helpful. Often, however, it is difficult to maintain a child or adolescent on lithium for extended periods because of the associated weight gain, exacerbation of acne, and hypothyroidism. If psychotic symptoms are present as part of the mania, treatment with an atypical antipsychotic agent is indicated and often is effective [65].

Most pediatric patients with pediatric bipolar disorder require combination pharmacotherapy for mood stabilization and symptom reduction, but the data on such treatment is limited [23,66]. In the only double-blind, placebo-controlled study of an atypical antipsychotic agent for the treatment of bipolar adolescents, quetiapine in combination with divalproex (n = 15) resulted in a greater reduction of manic symptoms than divalproex monotherapy (n = 15). This result suggests that the combination of a mood stabilizer and atypical antipsychotic agent is more effective than a mood stabilizer alone for the treatment of adolescent mania. In this study, quetiapine was titrated to a dose of 450 mg/day in 7 days and was well tolerated [18].

Most children with bipolar disorder have comorbid ADHD. In these patients, mood stabilization with a traditional mood stabilizer or an atypical antipsychotic agent is a necessary prerequisite before initiating stimulant medications [67]. A recent randomized, controlled trial of 40 bipolar children and adolescents with ADHD demonstrated that low-dose Dexedrine (Adderall XR) can be used safely and effectively for treatment of comorbid ADHD symptoms after the child's bipolar disorder symptoms are stabilized with divalproex [68]. Sustained-release psychostimulants may be more effective in reducing rebound symptoms in bipolar children and adolescents. A typical dose for a child with pediatric bipolar disorder and ADHD would be Concerta, 36 to 54 mg/day, or Adderall XR, 10 to 20 mg/day.

There is limited information regarding the treatment of depression in children and adolescents with bipolar disorder, and the role of antidepressants in the treatment of pediatric bipolar disorder depression is unclear. One retrospective study assessing treatment for depressed children and adolescents with bipolar disorder suggested that selective serotonin reuptake inhibitors (SSRIs) may be effective treatment for acute depression in bipolar children and adolescents without interfering with the acute antimanic effects of mood stabilizers. This report, however, also suggests that SSRIs may have mood destabilizing effects. Because too few subjects were being treated with mood stabilizers at the time that manic symptoms reemerged, the authors did not evaluate the protective effects of mood stabilizers in preventing the destabilizing effects [69]. This study indicated that depressive symptoms were 6.7 times more likely to improve when subjects received an SSRI than when they did not. In contrast, tricyclic antidepressants, stimulants, mood stabilizers, and typical antipsychotic agents were not significantly associated with improvement in depressive symptomatology. In this study, however, subjects receiving an SSRI were three times more likely to have developed manic symptoms at their next follow-up visit than subjects not taking an SSRI. Lamotrigine has been found to be effective in small case series of adolescents with bipolar disorder [70] and is an emerging option for the treatment of depression in these patients.

Summary

The identification and treatment of children and adolescents with a bipolar disorder is often challenging and difficult. Many of the psychotropic agents used to treat adults with bipolar disorder may also be used to treat children and adolescents with these disorders. Further controlled trials using combination pharmacotherapy in children and adolescents with bipolar disorders are needed to advance the field of pediatric bipolarity and provide optimal care for these patients. There are multiple ongoing trials of mood stabilizers and atypical antipsychotics that will provide important controlled data that are currently lacking in the field.

References

[1] Lewinsohn PM, Klein DN, Seeley JR. Bipolar disorders in a community sample of older adolescents: prevalence, phenomenology, comorbidity, and course. J Am Acad Child Adolesc Psychiatry 1995;34(4):454–63.
[2] Geller B, Luby J. Child and adolescent bipolar disorder: a review of the past 10 years. J Am Acad Child Adolesc Psychiatry 1997;36(9):1168–76.

[3] Geller B, Bolhofner K, Craney J, et al. Psychosocial functioning in a prepubertal and early adolescent bipolar disorder phenotype. J Am Acad Child Adolesc Psychiatry 2000;39(12): 1543–8.

[4] Weinberg WA, Brumback RA. Mania in childhood: case studies and literature review. Am J Dis Child 1976;130:380–5.

[5] Akiskal HS, Downs J, Jordan P, et al. Affective disorders in referred children and younger siblings of manic-depressives. Mode of onset and prospective course. Arch Gen Psychiatry 1985;42(10):996–1003.

[6] Wozniak J, Biederman J, Kiely K, et al. Mania-like symptoms suggestive of childhood-onset bipolar disorder in clinically referred children. J Am Acad Child Adolesc Psychiatry 1995; 34(7):867–76.

[7] Isaac G. Misdiagnosed bipolar disorder in adolescents in a special educational school and treatment program. J Clin Psychiatry 1992;53(4):133–6.

[8] Geller B, Sun K, Zimerman B, et al. Complex and rapid-cycling in bipolar children and adolescents: a preliminary study. J Affect Disord 1995;34(4):259–68.

[9] Geller B, Tillman R, Craney JL, et al. Four-year prospective outcome and natural history of mania in children with a prepubertal and early adolescent bipolar disorder phenotype. Arch Gen Psychiatry 2004;61(5):459–67.

[10] Geller B, Warner K, Williams M, et al. Prepubertal and young adolescent bipolarity versus ADHD: assessment and validity using the WASH-U-KSADS, CBCL, and TRF. Journal Affect Disord 1998;51:93–100.

[11] Faraone SV, Biederman J, Wozniak J, et al. Is comorbidity with ADHD a marker for juvenile-onset mania? J Am Acad Child Adolesc Psychiatry 1997;36(8):1046–55.

[12] West SA, McElroy SL, Strakowski SM, et al. Attention deficit hyperactivity disorder in adolescent mania. Am J Psychiatry 1995;152(2):271–3.

[13] Geller B, Williams M, Zimerman B, et al. Prepubertal and early adolescent bipolarity differentiate from ADHD by manic symptoms, grandiose delusions, ultra-rapid or ultradian cycling. J Affect Disord 1998;51:81–91.

[14] Kovacs M, Pollock M. Bipolar disorder and comorbid conduct disorder in childhood and adolescence. J Am Acad Child Adolesc Psychiatry 1995;34(6):715–23.

[15] Wilens TE, Biederman J, Kwon A, et al. Risk of substance use disorders in adolescents with bipolar disorder. J Am Acad Child Adolesc Psychiatry 2004;43(11):1380–6.

[16] Wozniak J, Biederman S, Faraone SV, et al. Mania in children with pervasive developmental disorder revisited. J Am Acad Child Adolesc Psychiatry 1997;36(11):1552–9, discussion 1559–60.

[17] Geller B, Cooper TB, Sun K, et al. Double-blind and placebo-controlled study of lithium for adolescent bipolar disorders with secondary substance dependency. J Am Acad Child Adolesc Psychiatry 1998;37(2):171–8.

[18] DelBello M, Schwiers M, Rosenberg H, et al. Quetiapine as adjunctive treatment for adolescent mania associated with bipolar disorder. J Am Acad Child Adolesc Psychiatry 2002;41(10):1216–23.

[19] Strober M, Morrell W, Lampert C, et al. Relapse following discontinuation of lithium maintenance therapy in adolescents with bipolar I illness: a naturalistic study. Am J Psychiatry 1990;147(4):457–61.

[20] Strober M. Mixed mania associated with tricyclic antidepressant therapy in prepubertal delusional depression: three cases. J Child Adolesc Psychopharmacol 1998;8(3):181–5.

[21] Kowatch RA, Suppes T, Carmody TJ, et al. Effect size of lithium, divalproex sodium and carbamazepine in children and adolescents with bipolar disorder. J Am Acad Child Adolesc Psychiatry 2000;39(6):713–20.

[22] Youngerman J, Canino IA. Lithium carbonate use in children and adolescents. A survey of the literature. Arch Gen Psychiatry 1978;35(2):216–24.

[23] Findling RL, McNamara NK, Gracious BL, et al. Combination lithium and divalproex sodium in pediatric bipolarity. J Am Acad Child Adolesc Psychiatry 2003;42(8):895–901.

[24] Wagner KD, Weller E, Biederman J, et al. An open-label trial of divalproex in children and adolescents with bipolar disorder. J Am Acad Child Adolesc Psychiatry 2002;41(10): 1224–30.

[25] West SA, Keck PEJ, McElroy SL, et al. Open trial of valproate in the treatment of adolescent mania. J Child Adolesc Psychopharmacol 1994;4:263–7.

[26] Papatheodorou G, Kutcher SP, Katic M, et al. The efficacy and safety of divalproex sodium in the treatment of acute mania in adolescents and young adults: an open clinical trial. J Clin Psychopharmacol 1995;15(2):110–6.

[27] Isojarvi JI, Laatikainen TJ, Pakarinen AJ, et al. Polycystic ovaries and hyperandrogenism in women taking valproate for epilepsy. N Engl J Med 1993;329(19):1383–8.

[28] Evans RW, Clay TH, Gualtieri CT. Carbamazepine in pediatric psychiatry. J Am Acad Child Adolesc Psychiatry 1987;26(1):2–8.

[29] Puente RM. The use of carbamazepine in the treatment of behavioral disorders in children. In: Birkmayer W, editor. Epileptic seizures—behavior—pain. Baltimore (MD): University Park Press; 1975. p. 243–52.

[30] O'Donovan C, Kusumakar V, Graves GR, et al. Menstrual abnormalities and polycystic ovary syndrome in women taking valproate for bipolar mood disorder. J Clin Psychiatry 2002;63(Apr):322–30.

[31] Nassir Ghaemi S, Ko JY, Katzow JJ. Oxcarbazepine treatment of refractory bipolar disorder: a retrospective chart review. Bipolar Disord 2002;4(1):70–4.

[32] Hummel B, Stampfer R, Grunze H, et al. Acute antimanic efficacy and safety of oxcarbazepine in and open trial with on-off-on design. Bipolar Disord 2001;3(Suppl 1):43.

[33] Kusumakar V, Yatham LN. An open study of lamotrigine in refractory bipolar depression. Psychiatry Res 1997;72:145–8.

[34] Messenheimer JA, Guberman AH. Rash with lamotrigine: dosing guidelines. Epilepsia 2000; 4:488.

[35] Messenheimer J. Efficacy and safety of lamotrigine in pediatric patients. J Child Neurol 2002; 17(Suppl 2):2S34–2S42.

[36] McElroy SL, Keck PE Jr. Pharmacologic agents for the treatment of acute bipolar mania. Biol Psychiatry 2000;48(6):539–57.

[37] Pande AC, Davidson JR, Jefferson JW, et al. Treatment of social phobia with gabapentin: a placebo-controlled study. J Clin Psychopharmacol 1999;19:341–8.

[38] Pande AC, Pollack MH, Crockatt J, et al. Placebo-controlled study of gabapentin treatment of panic disorder. J Clin Psychopharmacol 2000;20:467–71.

[39] Yatham LN, Kusumakar V, Calabrese JR, et al. Third generation anticonvulsants in bipolar disorder: a review of efficacy and summary of clinical recommendations. J Clin Psychiatry 2002;63:275–83.

[40] DelBello M, Kowatch R, Warner J, et al. Topiramate treatment for pediatric bipolar disorder: a retrospective chart review. J Child Adolesc Psychopharmacol 2002;12(4):323–30.

[41] Crawford P. An audit of topiramate use in a general neurology clinic. Seizure 1998;7:207–11.

[42] McElroy SL, Suppes T, Keck PE, et al. Open-label adjunctive topiramate in the treatment of bipolar disorders. Biol Psychiatry 2000;47(12):1025–33.

[43] Glick I, Murray S, Vasudevan P, et al. Treatment with atypical antipsychotics: new indications and new populations. J Psychiatr Res 2001;35:187–91.

[44] Kapur S, Remington G. Atypical antipsychotics: new directions and new challenges in the treatment of schizophrenia. Annu Rev Med 2001;52:503–17.

[45] Keck PJ, McElroy S, Arnold L. Bipolar disorder. Med Clin North Am 2001;85:645–61.

[46] Berk M, Ichim L, Brook S. Olanzapine compared to lithium in mania: a double-blind randomized controlled trial. Int Clin Psychopharmacol 1999;14:339–43.

[47] Tohen M, Sanger T, McElroy S, et al. Olanzapine versus placebo in the treatment of acute mania. Olanzapine HGEH Study Group. Am J Psychiatry 1999;156(May):702–9.

[48] Tohen M, Jacobs TG, Grundy SL, et al. Efficacy of olanzapine in acute bipolar mania: a double-blind, placebo-controlled study. Arch Gen Psychiatry 2000;57(9):841–9.

[49] Segal J, Berk M, Brook S. Risperidone compared with both lithium and haloperidol in mania: a double-blind randomized controlled trial. Clin Neuropharmacol 1998;21:176–80.

[50] Sachs GS, Grossman F, Ghaemi SN, et al. Combination of a mood stabilizer with risperidone or haloperidol for treatment of acute mania: a double-blind, placebo-controlled comparison of efficacy and safety. Am J Psychiatry 2002;159(7):1146–54.

[51] Keck PE Jr, Marcus R, Tourkodimitris S, et al. A placebo-controlled, double-blind study of the efficacy and safety of aripiprazole in patients with acute bipolar mania. Am J Psychiatry 2003;160(9):1651–8.

[52] Keck P, Ice K, Ziprasidone MSG. A 3-week, double-blind, randomized trial of ziprasidone in the acute treatment of mania. Presented at the 40th annual meeting NCDEU. Boca Raton, FL, May 30–June 2, 2000.

[53] Keck PJ, Reeves K, Harrigan E. Ziprasidone in the short-term treatment of patients with schizoaffective disorder: results from two double-blind, placebo-controlled, multicenter studies. J Clin Psychopharmacol 2001;21:27–35.

[54] Kowatch RA, Suppes T, Gilfillan SK, et al. Clozapine treatment of children and adolescents with bipolar disorder and schizophrenia: a clinical case series. J Child Adolesc Psychopharmacol 1995;5(4):241–53.

[55] Frazier J, Meyer M, Biederman J, et al. Risperidone treatment for juvenile bipolar disorder: a retrospective chart review. J Am Acad Child Adolesc Psychiatry 1999;38:960–5.

[56] Soutullo C, Sorter M, Foster K, et al. Olanzapine in the treatment of adolescent acute mania: a report of seven cases. J Affect Disord 1999;53:279–83.

[57] Khouzam HR, El-Gabalawi F. Treatment of bipolar I disorder in an adolescent with olanzapine. J Child Adolesc Psychopharmacol 2000;10:147–51.

[58] Chang K, Ketter T. Mood stabilizer augmentation with olanzapine in acutely manic children. J Child Adolesc Psychopharmacol 2000;10:45–9.

[59] Ratzoni G, Gothelf D, Brand-Gothelf A, et al. Weight gain associated with olanzapine and risperidone in adolescent patients: a comparative prospective study. J Am Acad Child Adolesc Psychiatry 2002;4:337–43.

[60] Clark C, Burge MR. Diabetes mellitus associated with atypical anti-psychotic medications. Diabetes Technol Ther 2003;5(4):669–83.

[61] Lebovitz HE. Metabolic consequences of atypical antipsychotic drugs. Psychiatr Q 2003; 74(3):277–90.

[62] American Diabetes Association. American Psychiatric Association. Consensus development conference on antipsychotic drugs and obesity and diabetes. Diabetes Care 2004;27(2): 596–601.

[63] Weiden P. Ziprasidone: a new atypical antipsychotic. J Psychiatr Pract 2001;145–53.

[64] Blair J, Scahill L, State M, et al. Electrocardiographic changes in children and adolescents treated with ziprasidone: a prospective study. J Am Acad Child Adolesc Psychiatry 2005; 44(1):73–9.

[65] Kowatch RA, DelBello MP. The use of mood stabilizers and atypical antipsychotics in children and adolescents with bipolar disorders. CNS Spectr 2003;8(4):273–80.

[66] Kowatch RA, Sethuraman G, Hume JH, et al. Combination pharmacotherapy in children and adolescents with bipolar disorder. Biol Psychiatry 2003;53(11):978–84.

[67] Biederman J, Mick E, Prince J, et al. Systematic chart review of the pharmacologic treatment of comorbid attention deficit hyperactivity disorder in youth with bipolar disorder. J Child Adolesc Psychopharmacol 1999;9(4):247–56.

[68] Scheffer R, Kowatch R, Carmody T, et al. A randomized placebo-controlled trial of Adderall for symptoms of comorbid ADHD in pediatric bipolar disorder following mood stabilization with divalproex sodium. Am J Psychiatry 2005;162:58–64.

[69] Biederman J, Mick E, Spencer TJ, et al. Therapeutic dilemmas in the pharmacotherapy of bipolar depression in the young. J Child Adolesc Psychopharmacol 2000;10(3):185–92.

[70] Carandang CG, Maxwell DJ, Robbins DR, et al. Lamotrigine in adolescent mood disorders. J Am Acad Child Adolesc Psychiatry 2003;42(7):750–1.

ELSEVIER
SAUNDERS

Psychiatr Clin N Am
28 (2005) 399–414

PSYCHIATRIC
CLINICS
OF NORTH AMERICA

Mood-stabilizing Drugs: Are Their Neuroprotective Aspects Clinically Relevant?

Diane C. Lagace, PhD, Amelia J. Eisch, PhD*

*Department of Psychiatry, University of Texas Southwestern Medical Center,
5323 Harry Hines Boulevard, Dallas, TX 75390, USA*

The 1949 report of lithium's efficacy in the treatment of bipolar disorder and its approval for treatment in 1970 marked a new era in pharmacotherapy for this chronic, severe illness [1,2]. Understanding how a simple cation effectively attenuates abnormal mood swings surely would lead to intelligent drug design, and the myriad of new treatments that were predicted to emerge from this approach would be of enormous help to the 1% to 2% of the population affected by bipolar disorder [3,4]. Fifty years later, however, it is notable that clinically effective drugs for bipolar disorder—lithium, a variety of anticonvulsant drugs such as valproic acid, carbamazepine, and lamotrigine, and certain antipsychotics [5–8]—emerged serendipitously, not from any solid evidence about the neural actions of the drugs.

Chance drug discovery has played an important role in the treatment and understanding of the neural basis for other psychiatric disorders, such as major depressive disorder [9]. Indeed, discovery of the second-generation antidepressants opened broad avenues for studying the neural under-pinnings of depression. In the case of mood-stabilizing drugs, however, solid hypotheses about a common neural mechanism for clinically effective drugs have evaded researchers for many years. Recently a broad net cast across effective mood-stabilizing drugs presented a candidate commonality: all of these drugs have neuroprotective characteristics [10–13]. From this com-monality a reasonable hypothesis has emerged that the neuroprotective aspects of mood-stabilizing drugs underlie their clinical efficacy. In

This work was supported by a Young Investigator Award from the National Alliance for Research on Schizophrenia and Depression (AE) and by grants from the National Institute of Health (AE) and the Canadian Institute for Health Research (DL).

* Corresponding author.

E-mail address: amelia.eisch@southwestern.edu (A.J. Eisch).

particular, it is proposed that the neuroprotective actions of mood-stabilizing drugs are mediated by their neurotrophic, nerve-nourishing effects. Although endogenous neurotrophic factors, such as nerve growth factor and brain-derived neurotrophic factor, traditionally have been viewed in terms of their ability to increase cell survival by providing trophic support, their survival effects are also mediated by the inhibition of apoptosis, such as through inhibition of the cell-death cascades. In addition to cell survival and prevention of cell death, it is postulated that mood-stabilizing drugs act to encourage adult neurogenesis, the birth of new cells in the adult brain [10,14,15]. The possibility that mood-stabilizing drugs mediate their clinical effects through neuroprotection, neurotropism, and neurogenesis raises several intriguing questions. Is bipolar disorder marked by neuronal injury? Should rationally designed drugs for future use in bipolar disorder specifically target neuroprotective cascades in the brain? Might such drugs find a wider use, for example in treating classic neuro-degenerative disorders such as Huntington's disease?

The neuroprotective hypothesis of mood-stabilizing drugs has a significant amount of support when viewed from a biochemical perspective. The biochemical pathways through which drugs such as lithium and valproic acid are thought to mediate their neuroprotective effects are well studied, and readers are referred to several recent and excellent reviews for detailed explanation of these cascades [11,12,16–19]. In addition, many studies using in vitro cell culture and in vivo laboratory animals, as well as imaging studies in humans, support the theory that the neuroprotective aspect of mood-stabilizing drugs is important for their clinical efficacy [20–28]. In the determined push to find commonality in the diverse medications effective for treating mood disorders, however, several gaps in knowledge and inconsistencies have emerged that deserve consideration. For example, in vitro evidence of neuroprotection comes from brain regions not apparently damaged in the brains of bipolar patients, such as the cerebellum. In addition, a dearth of good animal models of bipolar disorder place the onus on human research to show that bipolar disorder is marked by cell or volume loss and that those changes are normalized by mood-stabilizing drugs. Even imaging work in humans is problematic in this regard, because many studies have small numbers of patients, and only a few have a longitudinal design. Finally, many studies have emphasized similarities among drugs, instead of important differences. Given the likely diversity of the disorder itself, such differences should be carefully examined for their potential contribution to the hypothesis that aspects of these drugs un-related to their neuroprotective qualities may be clinically relevant.

This article summarizes the current evidence that mood-stabilizing drugs are neuroprotective and evaluates the hypothesis that these effects could mediate their therapeutic efficacy in bipolar disorder. It also highlights gaps in the hypothesis that mood-stabilizing drugs are therapeutic in bipolar disorder because of their neuroprotective properties. By careful evaluation of the neuroprotective hypothesis concerning mood-stabilizing drugs, the authors hope to encourage identification of important targets of current mood-stabilizing drugs. That knowledge could be used to design more specific and efficacious medications.

The neuroprotective properties of mood-stabilizing drugs in cultured cells

Given the complexity of bipolar disorder, it may be striking to a clinician that the neuroprotective hypothesis of mood-stabilizing drugs received much of its initial and strongest support from in vitro work done on cultured cells. Indeed, ample in vitro evidence demonstrates the ability of lithium, valproic acid, carbamazepine, and lamotrigine to protect neural cells from a variety of insults, including excitotoxicity, heat-shock, and nutrient or mineral deprivation [20,23,29–39]. These studies have been central to the elucidation of the biochemical pathways used by mood-stabilizing drugs. Two aspects of these in vitro models may not be clinically relevant, however. First, the in vitro insults typically result in cell death, which has not yet been clearly observed in the human bipolar brain. Second, many of these studies typically use either immortalized cell lines or primary cerebellar granule cells that come from the cerebellum, which is thought not to be affected in bipolar disorder. Therefore, although these studies are a necessary component to future drug design for bipolar disorder, caution is encouraged in interpreting their results too broadly.

Three aspects of these in vitro studies deserve closer attention, because their examination may reveal important angles for future drug design. First, although there is mounting evidence that the mood-stabilizing drugs are neuroprotective in culture, the neuroprotective effects of mood stabilizers do not seem to occur in all brain cells. For example, proliferation in response to lithium has differing effects in neuronal cells and astrocytes. In serum-deprived neurons, lithium induces proliferation, whereas in astrocytes lithium inhibits DNA synthesis and induces a G2/M cell cycle arrest [40]. This effect may be beneficial when using lithium for a treatment against a disease such as stroke, where it is optimal to favor neural repair and reduce reactive gliosis. Second, mood stabilizers do not protect against all forms of insult in an in vitro system. For example, lithium has been demonstrated not to be neuroprotective against apoptotic signaling induced by activation of the Fas death domain–containing receptor [41]. A comparison of the effect of lithium on a variety of insults in cerebellar granule cells showed that lithium is protective against apoptosis induced by antipsychotic treatment, aging of the culture, or growth in low-potassium concentrations but is ineffective in preventing apoptosis from many other insults, such as the addition of protein kinase inhibitor or nitric oxide donor [31]. Third, in vitro studies have demonstrated that a neuroprotective effect identified for one mood stabilizer may not be common to all mood stabilizers. In ouabain-induced cell death and in colchicine-induced cell death, lithium has been shown to be neuroprotective, but valproic acid is not [36,42]. In a model of staurosporine- and heat-shock–induced apoptosis in SH-SY5Y cells overexpressing glycogen synthase kinase 3β, valproic acid or lamotrigine is neuroprotective, but carbamazepine is not [35]. Similarly, in serum-deprived SH-SY5Y cells, valproic acid induces neurite outgrowth and suppresses cell death, whereas varying concentrations of lithium, carbamazepine, and lamotrigine do not have this effect [43]. Together these studies suggest that different mood stabilizers may mediate their neuroprotective effects through distinct mechanisms. This possibility is clearly an important avenue for future study.

Because debate continues about whether the bipolar brain has frank cell death, it is instructive to consider the few studies that have addressed the neurotrophic and neurogenic effects of mood stabilizers. In general, these studies have assessed neuron proliferation, neurite outgrowth, regeneration, and differentiation. In sensory neurons lithium, valproic acid, and carbamazepine have a common effect of increasing growth cone formation, leading to a spreading of the neuron and a shorter neuronal axon [27]. More recently, however, this effect has not been seen with the mood stabilizer lamotrigine [44]. In undifferentiated primary cultures of rat cerebellar granule cells and cerebral cortical cells, lithium treatment for a minimum of 2 to 4 days increased proliferation. In the case of the cerebral cortical neurons, 90% of these diving cells were colocalized with the neuroblast or progenitor cell marker nestin, leading to the conclusion that lithium treatment induces neuronal progenitor cell proliferation [45]. In agreement with this finding, others have demonstrated that lithium treatment decreases apoptosis of nestin-positive progenitors in telencephalic neuroepithelial cells from mouse embryos [46]. Recently, lithium has been shown to induce proliferation and neuronal differentiation of rat hippocampal progenitor cells regardless of whether the cells were grown in the presence or absence of a mitogen [26]. Like lithium, valproic acid treatment has been shown to induce neurogenesis in vitro, specifically inducing neurite growth, cell reemergence, and the formation of mature neurons in embryonic cortical cells [25]. Similarly, valproic acid treatment has been demonstrated to promote proliferation of embryonic rat cortical or human striatal primordial stem cells and to enhance differentiation of neurons that have a γ-aminobutyric acid (GABA)ergic phenotype [47]. Lithium also was demonstrated to enhance proliferation of the cortical progenitors, but treatment with carbamazepine was ineffective [47]. Together these studies support the hypothesis that lithium and valproic acid are able to induce proliferation of progenitor cells in vitro. Although it is reasonable to generalize these effects to state that mood-stabilizing drugs are neurogenic, it is also important to pursue the differences noted (eg, why carbamazepine or lamotrigine may not be as potent in induced neurogenesis as lithium and valproic acid).

These in vitro results suggest a tantalizing link between neuroprotection and neurogenesis and mood-stabilizing drugs and represent the bulk of research to determine mechanisms by which these drugs have these neuro-protective properties. The relevance of the effects of these drugs in vitro to the treatment of bipolar disorder in patients is not clear, however. Because bipolar disorder is not thought to be marked by frank cell death, it is likely that neuroprotection and neurogenesis are not the only neural underpinnings of the therapeutic effects of these medications. Because some of the neuro-protective effects are not common to all mood stabilizers, these effects may not be important for the efficacy of these medications. Alternatively, different mood-stabilizing drugs are effective in different populations of patients with bipolar disorder, and it is possible that these differences may account for the unique response profile of each medication and could be of therapeutic advantage. Bipolar disorder, like schizophrenia, may actually be a collection of disorders, each sensitive to a particular pharmacotherapy. Indeed the diverse presentation of bipolar disorder—periods of mania, hypomania, mixed states, major depression or depressive mixed states [48]—has led to a complex decision tree for treatment. For example, the most recent American Psychiatric Association practice guidelines for the treatment of patients with bipolar disorder recommend acute mania therapy be initiated with lithium or valproic acid or an antipsychotic, alone or in combination, depending on the severity of the illness and presentation of symptoms [49]. For acute bipolar disorder depressive episodes, initial treatment with either lithium or lamotrigine is recommended [49]. Given the relative success of such a decision tree, a future goal for in vitro assessment of mood-stabilizing drugs is to identify neural and biochemical commonalities within these drugs that might help explain why certain drugs are more appropriate in certain clinical situations. In addition, to determine whether the neuroprotective aspects of mood-stabilizing drugs are important to a disease state, studies also need to assess the neuroprotective and neurogenic effects of these medications in vivo in animal models.

The neuroprotective or neurogenic properties of mood stabilizers in animals

The largest hurdle in assessing the neuroprotective or neurogenic properties of mood-stabilizing drugs in animals is finding an appropriate animal model for bipolar disorder. As many excellent reviews have summa-rized, the difficultly in modeling bipolar disorder in animals is that no cur-rent models are able to depict the oscillating pattern of mood, the hallmark of bipolar disorder [9,50,51]. Lacking the ability to model mood swings, several models have instead focused on mimicking either a depressive or a manic phenotype. Models of mania in laboratory animals include sleep deprivation, neurodevelopmental brain lesion, kindling, and psychostimu-lant-induced hyperactivity; the last is the standard model used to screen antimanic drugs [9,51]. Models of depression include chronic stress, early life stress, tail suspension, learned helplessness, and the forced swim test, with the last being the standard model to screen antidepressant drugs [9,52].

Most of these models have both face validity (the commonality of behaviors between the model and human disorder) and predictive validity (the degree to which the model responds to currently used mood stabilizers). More recently, models have been developed from a construct validity starting point, in which the model attempts to recapitulate the causation or pathology associated with the disease. For example, mania was discovered to be associated with decreased activity of the sodium- and potassium-activated ATP membrane pump. From this discovery, a model of mania has been developed in which a specific inhibitor of this pump, ouabain, is given to rodents. The hyperactivity that developed from ouabain exposure can be prevented with 1 week of lithium treatment [53–55]. Moreover, inducible transgenic mouse technology has allowed the development of new models based on constructive validity. For example, a mouse in which the glucocorticoid receptor is overexpressed has been proposed as a model for increased emotional lability and possibly bipolar disorder [56]. Although no model has yet to fully model bipolar disorder in rodents, these models provide valuable tools with which to evaluate current therapies. There is significant excitement in the field that animal models still in development will be instrumental in uncovering the mechanism of actions for mood stabilizers and thus lead to improved drug design.

Given the numerous publications touting the potential neuroprotective and neurogenic actions of mood-stabilizing drugs, it is surprising that to date only one study has evaluated this hypothesis in an animal model of depression or mania. The chronic restraint -stress model of depression has been shown previously to produce a striking loss of dendritic arborization in hippocampal neurons. A recent study showed that lithium is effective in preventing this stress-induced loss of dendrites [28]. The inhibition of stress-induced changes in dendritic length was associated with increased glutamatergic activity, suggesting that lithium's effects are mediated by decreasing excitotoxicity. In addition, lithium had no effect on dendritic length in animals that were not stressed, suggesting that the effects of lithium are specific to a damaged neural environment. This latter point is especially intriguing, given the efficacy of mood-stabilizing drugs to prevent or attenuate injury in animal models of stroke, ischemia, and other models of neurodegenerative diseases [57–66]. Such studies provide support for the assertion that mood-stabilizing drugs may be valuable in the treatment or prevention of stroke, Huntington's disease, or Alzheimer's disease [12]. This novel application for mood-stabilizing drugs certainly deserves further study. It is clear, however, that the rodent models of bipolar disorder, however imperfect, should be the focus of future efforts to examine more closely the hypothesis that mood-stabilizing drugs are indeed neuroprotective or neurogenic.

Given the imperfection of animal models of bipolar disorder, an alternative strategy to evaluate the neural mechanisms of mood-stabilizing drugs is to examine the effects of these medications in healthy, naïve rodents. This approach is common with other psychotropic drugs, such as antidepressants and antipsychotics [52], and has been used recently to demonstrate the neurogenic effect of lithium. Two to 4 weeks of lithium have been shown to increase the number of newly formed hippocampal cells in the adult rat and mouse [24,67]. A shorter 2-day exposure to lithium did not influence the number of new hippocampal cells. As with antidepressant treatment, lithium's neurogenic time course is tantalizingly similar to the time course for clinical efficacy [68]. Lithium's impact seems to be limited to increased proliferation, because studies have shown that chronic exposure does not influence the fate of the cells (eg, only the number of cells is different, not the proportion of dividing cells that mature into neurons). Lithium's ability to increase neurogenesis in animals is age dependent; in older rats, 14 days of lithium treatment does not alter the number of adult-generated cells that express a mature neuronal maker [69]. This finding is interesting in light of the relative paucity of research done on the clinical efficacy of mood-stabilizing drugs in later life. Although these studies in naïve rodents underscore the neurogenic potential of lithium, no studies have examined the ability of mood-stabilizing drugs to decrease basal levels of cell death in the naïve brain. Such studies would strengthen the neuroprotective hypothesis of mood-stabilizing drugs.

An important commonality of the three studies examining the neurogenic effect of lithium is that the method of detecting new cells—multiple injections of the S-phase marker BrdU instead of a single injection—obscures lithium's possible impact on the proliferation or survival of the new cells. Given evidence that lithium is neuroprotective, it is possible that lithium increases the number of new cells by preventing their death rather than by stimulating their proliferation. Indeed, recently the antidepressant fluoxetine has been shown to induce proliferation as well as increase cell death [70]. This distinction would be revealing in regards to lithium's neural mechanism, and therefore additional studies of lithium's neurogenic effects with greater temporal resolution are warranted. Studies that have been performed using valproic acid are instructive in this regard. A single BrdU injection given to rats after 6 weeks of treatment with valproic acid did not alter the number of proliferating cells in the hippocampus [25]. When the single BrdU injection was given before 6 weeks of valproic acid, however, there was a significant increase in the number of labeled dividing cells. Although the fate of these surviving cells was not quantified, and therefore the extent to which valproic acid stimulates neurogenesis is not known, this study suggests that valproic acid's effects may indeed be neuroprotective, not neurogenic per se.

Overall, research on the effects of lithium or valproic acid supports the hypothesis that mood-stabilizing drugs induce neuroprotection. Once it has been established whether these medications alter neurogenesis, it will be interesting to translate this work into animal models of bipolar disorder and to try to establish whether increasing neurogenesis is required and is associated with treatment effects in these models. This approach has been demonstrated recently in the case of antidepressants in an animal model of depression [71–73]. It will also be necessary for future work to include female rodents in models of mood disorders, because these medications are used in both male and female patients. Despite the need for animal research to assess the effects of these drugs, there are no guarantees that any models will be able to predict human response accurately. For example, despite a wealth of research demonstrating increases in neurogenesis occurring in animal models of epilepsy, there is little evidence of increased neurogenesis in patients with epilepsy as assessed in tissue dissected from intractable epileptics [74].

The neuroprotective and neurogenic properties of mood stabilizers in humans

Although in vitro and laboratory animal studies are indispensable in the exploration of the neural mechanisms of mood-stabilizing drugs, determining whether the neuroprotective or neurogenic properties are important for mood-stabilizing drugs requires evidence that patients with bipolar disorder have abnormal neuropathology and that correcting these abnormalities is associated with a positive clinical response. Post-mortem analysis and, more recently, structural and functional brain imaging studies have helped to compile a growing compendium of the pathophysiology of bipolar disorder [reviewed in 13,22,75,76]. In general, functional imaging suggests that bipolar disorder is marked by alterations in activation as well as by abnormalities in membranes and second-messenger metabolism within the cortical and subcortical regions. To assess the neuroprotective hypothesis of mood-stabilizing drugs, this section highlights studies suggesting that bipolar disorder may be associated with alterations in brain volume or brain cell number.

The excitement about the possibility that the neuroprotective effects of mood stabilizers might be associated with clinical efficacy arose following reports suggesting that patients treated with lithium show an increase in gray matter. This prospective volumetric study of bipolar patients receiving lithium therapy for 4 weeks demonstrated that lithium increased the total gray matter content, which the authors suggested was a result of the medication's increasing the volume of the neuropil, the axonal and dendritic fibers within the cortex gray matter volume [77]. A cross-sectional study has confirmed these results, finding an increase in total gray matter volume in lithium-treated patients compared with untreated patients and healthy controls [21]. The increase in gray matter did not occur in healthy volunteers treated with lithium, suggesting that lithium has specific effects in patients with bipolar disorder [19]. Moreover, in a study of bipolar twins and their co-twins, a positive correlation has been reported between frontal gray matter volume and use of lithium therapy [78]. More recent work has examined whether these medication effects are specific to certain subregions of the brain. Preliminary findings suggest that there are prominent alterations in gray matter volumes in the hippocampus, caudate, and prefrontal cortex [19].

It has also been reported that unmedicated bipolar patients have decreased left anterior cingulate gray matter volumes when compared with healthy control subjects and with bipolar patients treated with lithium monotherapy [79]. Although still preliminary, these findings support the hypothesis that mood-stabilizing drugs are neuroprotective in suggesting that bipolar disorder is marked by a decline in gray matter volume, and that lithium is associated with increased gray matter volume within certain brain regions. Future studies are now needed to identify whether other mood stabilizers, such as valproic acid, have similar effects.

These findings suggest that patients with bipolar disorder have an associated decline in gray matter volume. There are, however, many conflicting reports about whether bipolar disorder is associated with alterations in gray matter volume, as assessed by magnetic resonance imaging (MRI) and magnetic resonance spectroscopy. When examining patients with bipolar disorder, many studies report no significant alterations in global gray matter volume [78,80–86], and four studies report decreased cortical gray matter volume [87–90]. Upon examining reductions in gray matter in specific cortical regions of patients with bipolar disorder, many studies report the consistent result of decreased gray matter volume within the prefrontal cortex [87,91–94]. The meaning of these volumetric changes is difficult to assess, because they could be caused by a variety of factors, including neurodevelopmental abnormalities associated with bipolar disorder, changes in regional blood flow, changes in the neuron or glial cell number, and trait- or disease-state–related factors [76]. To decipher these possibilities, current research is being developed that assesses these alterations in longitudinal studies, in individuals who do not display clinical symptoms but are at a higher risk for the development of bipolar disorder, and in studies using the combination of MRI with post-mortem studies to elucidate cell number and shape.

Neuropathologic investigations have already identified alterations in neuronal cell size and number and in glial cell number within the cortex [13]. When assessing the total number of neurons across all cortical regions, two studies report no differences in patients with bipolar disorder compared with controls [95,96]. Similar to the neuroimaging work, however, further analysis of regional differences within the brain suggests reductions in neuronal densities in a subset of cortical layers [96–98]. Morphologic analysis suggests a reduction in the number of nonpyramidal inhibitory GABAergic neurons and in the number of pyramidal excitatory glutamatergic neurons in patients with bipolar disorder [96,97]. An increase in neuron number has been identified in certain subregions of the brain of patients with bipolar disorder, such as the locus coeruleus [99]. The decreases and increases in number of neurons within different areas of the brain in patients with bipolar disorder has been suggested to be in agreement with the complex characteristics of the illness: alterations in affect, in cognition, and in neuroendocrine systems and circadian rhythms [13].

Similar to the region-specific alterations in neuronal cell number, there are reports of region-specific alterations in glial number. One study reports a striking 41% reduction in the number of glial cells in the medial prefrontal cortex in patients with familiar bipolar disorder [95]. Also, patients with bipolar disorder who are not treated with valproic acid or lithium seem to have fewer glial cells in the amygdala, a brain region important in emotional processing and emotional memory [100]. In contrast, glial cell numbers seem to be normal within all layers of the anterior cingulate cortex [97], the dorsal lateral prefrontal cortex [96], and the sensorimotor cortex [95] in bipolar disorder. Although the clinical implications of fewer glial cells in the medial prefrontal and amygdala are unknown, the region-specific nature of the decrease emphasizes that this area warrants further research.

Despite the evidence that bipolar disorder is associated with reduction in number, density, or size of neurons and glial cells, bipolar disorder is distinct from classical neurodegenerative diseases, such as Huntington's disease, as reviewed by Rajkowska [13]. The most obvious difference between bipolar disorder and classic neurodegenerative diseases is that there is a lack of gliosis in bipolar disorder; no studies to date have reported increased glial cell density or glial hypertrophy. The absence of glial pathology suggests that the brain is not actively responding to the ongoing reduction of neurons in patients with bipolar disorder. Moreover, it is unknown whether the cell pathology associated with bipolar disorder occurs before onset of the illness or whether these changes are primarily associated with manic or depressed episodes.

Summary

The possibility that there may be subtypes of bipolar disorder and the slow progress in understanding the therapeutic mechanism for approved mood-stabilizing drugs make the challenges of intelligent drug design seem daunting. Nonetheless, the numerous shortcomings in current pharmaco-therapy underscore the need to develop novel therapies. There are significant problems with currently approved mood-stabilizing drugs:

1. Up to 40% of patients fail to respond to monotherapy with either lithium or valproic acid.
2. Common use of polypharmacotherapy increases the side effects associated with treatment [101].
3. Treatment must continue for weeks to months for therapeutic effects to be greater than placebo.
4. Up to 60% of patients will discontinue therapy, which is somewhat attributable to unwanted side effects [102].

Thus, it is critical that new medications without these problems be developed for bipolar disorder. The hypothesis that mood-stabilizing drugs are neuroprotective is an important first step in new drug development.

To determine if the clinical efficacy of mood-stabilizing drugs is dependent on the neuroprotective or neurogenic properties of these medications, greater strides need to be made in relating findings from cell culture and animal models to human imaging and pathology. Mounting evidence supports the neuroprotective and neurogenic properties of lithium and valproic acid in a variety of cell-culture models. It is important for clinical, biochemical, and in vitro differences between these medications to be examined, not ignored, because these differences may reveal critical distinctions between the neural mechanisms of these drugs. Continuation of the in vitro work will aid in the understanding of the mechanism by which these drugs are neuroprotective, but such studies do not advance the understanding of whether these effects are critical for the clinical efficacy of these medications. In attempting to understand the in vivo effects of these medications, a variety of evidence supports the neuroprotective and neurogenic aspects of lithium and valproic acid in healthy rodents and animal models of gross brain insult. More work needs to be done to assess whether these effects occur in animal models for bipolar disorder. The proof of principle for supporting the claim that the neuroprotective or neurogenic properties are important clinically will come from longitudinal clinical studies that compare brain morphology and function before and during treatment. If enough evidence supports the hypothesis that the neuroprotective and neurogenic properties of mood-stabilizing drugs are important for their clinical efficacy, new medications that are more efficacious and have fewer side effects will be designed based on this discovery.

References

[1] Manji HK, Moore GJ, Chen G. Lithium at 50: have the neuroprotective effects of this unique cation been overlooked? Biol Psychiatry 1999;46(7):929–40.
[2] Cade J. Lithium salts in the treatment of psychotic symptoms. Med J Aust 1949;36:349–52.
[3] Kessler RC, McGonagle KA, Zhao S, et al. Lifetime and 12-month prevalence of DSM-III-R psychiatric disorders in the United States. Results from the National Comorbidity Survey. Arch Gen Psychiatry 1994;51(1):8–19.
[4] Weissman MM, Bland RC, Canino GJ, et al. Cross-national epidemiology of major depression and bipolar disorder. JAMA 1996;276(4):293–9.
[5] Hirschfeld RM, Vornik LA. Recognition and diagnosis of bipolar disorder. J Clin Psychiatry 2004;65(Suppl 15):5–9.
[6] Lennkh C, Simhandl C. Current aspects of valproate in bipolar disorder. Int Clin Psychopharmacol 2000;15(1):1–11.
[7] Yatham LN. Newer anticonvulsants in the treatment of bipolar disorder. J Clin Psychiatry 2004;65(Suppl 10):28–35.
[8] Schatzberg AF. Employing pharmacologic treatment of bipolar disorder to greatest effect. J Clin Psychiatry 2004;65(Suppl 15):15–20.
[9] Nestler EJ, Gould E, Manji H, et al. Preclinical models: status of basic research in depression. Biol Psychiatry 2002;52(6):503–28.
[10] Manji HK, Moore GJ, Chen G. Clinical and preclinical evidence for the neurotrophic effects of mood stabilizers: implications for the pathophysiology and treatment of manic-depressive illness. Biol Psychiatry 2000;48(8):740–54.

[11] Brunello N. Mood stabilizers: protecting the mood, protecting the brain. J Affect Disord 2004;79(Suppl 1):S15–20.
[12] Rowe MK, Chuang DM. Lithium neuroprotection: molecular mechanisms and clinical implications. Expert Rev Mol Med 2004;6(21):1–18.
[13] Rajkowska G. Cell pathology in mood disorders. Semin Clin Neuropsychiatry 2002;7(4): 281–92.
[14] Eisch AJ. Adult neurogenesis: implications for psychiatry. Prog Brain Res 2002;138: 315–42.
[15] Coyle JT, Duman RS. Finding the intracellular signaling pathways affected by mood disorder treatments. Neuron 2003;38(2):157–60.
[16] Bauer M, Alda M, Priller J, et al. Implications of the neuroprotective effects of lithium for the treatment of bipolar and neurodegenerative disorders. Pharmacopsychiatry 2003; 36(Suppl 3):S250–4.
[17] Li X, Ketter TA, Frye MA. Synaptic, intracellular, and neuroprotective mechanisms of anticonvulsants: are they relevant for the treatment and course of bipolar disorders? J Affect Disord 2002;69(1–3):1–14.
[18] Quiroz JA, Singh J, Gould TD, et al. Emerging experimental therapeutics for bipolar disorder: clues from the molecular pathophysiology. Mol Psychiatry 2004;9(8):756–76.
[19] Gould TD, Quiroz JA, Singh J, et al. Emerging experimental therapeutics for bipolar disorder: insights from the molecular and cellular actions of current mood stabilizers. Mol Psychiatry 2004;9(8):734–55.
[20] Mora A, Gonzalez-Polo RA, Fuentes JM, et al. Different mechanisms of protection against apoptosis by valproate and Li^+. Eur J Biochem 1999;266(3):886–91.
[21] Sassi RB, Nicoletti M, Brambilla P, et al. Increased gray matter volume in lithium-treated bipolar disorder patients. Neurosci Lett 2002;329(2):243–5.
[22] Strakowski SM, Delbello MP, Adler CM. The functional neuroanatomy of bipolar disorder: a review of neuroimaging findings. Mol Psychiatry 2005;10(1):105–16.
[23] Bown CD, Wang JF, Young LT. Attenuation of N-methyl-D-aspartate-mediated cytoplasmic vacuolization in primary rat hippocampal neurons by mood stabilizers. Neuroscience 2003;117(4):949–55.
[24] Chen G, Rajkowska G, Du F, et al. Enhancement of hippocampal neurogenesis by lithium. J Neurochem 2000;75(4):1729–34.
[25] Hao Y, Creson T, Zhang L, et al. Mood stabilizer valproate promotes ERK pathway-dependent cortical neuronal growth and neurogenesis. J Neurosci 2004;24(29):6590–9.
[26] Kim JS, Chang MY, Yu IT, et al. Lithium selectively increases neuronal differentiation of hippocampal neural progenitor cells both in vitro and in vivo. J Neurochem 2004;89(2): 324–36.
[27] Williams RS, Cheng L, Mudge AW, et al. A common mechanism of action for three mood-stabilizing drugs. Nature 2002;417(6886):292–5.
[28] Wood GE, Young LT, Reagan LP, et al. Stress-induced structural remodeling in hippocampus: prevention by lithium treatment. Proc Natl Acad Sci U S A 2004;101(11): 3973–8.
[29] Kopnisky KL, Chalecka-Franaszek E, Gonzalez-Zulueta M, et al. Chronic lithium treatment antagonizes glutamate-induced decrease of phosphorylated CREB in neurons via reducing protein phosphatase 1 and increasing MEK activities. Neuroscience 2003; 116(2):425–35.
[30] Hashimoto R, Hough C, Nakazawa T, et al. Lithium protection against glutamate excitotoxicity in rat cerebral cortical neurons: involvement of NMDA receptor inhibition possibly by decreasing NR2B tyrosine phosphorylation. J Neurochem 2002;80(4):589–97.
[31] Nonaka S, Katsube N, Chuang DM. Lithium protects rat cerebellar granule cells against apoptosis induced by anticonvulsants, phenytoin and carbamazepine. J Pharmacol Exp Ther 1998;286(1):539–47.

[32] Grignon S, Levy N, Couraud F, et al. Tyrosine kinase inhibitors and cycloheximide inhibit Li + protection of cerebellar granule neurons switched to non-depolarizing medium. Eur J Pharmacol 1996;315(1):111–4.

[33] Li R, El-Mallakh RS. A novel evidence of different mechanisms of lithium and valproate neuroprotective action on human SY5Y neuroblastoma cells: caspase-3 dependency. Neurosci Lett 2000;294(3):147–50.

[34] Yuan PX, Huang LD, Jiang YM, et al. The mood stabilizer valproic acid activates mitogen-activated protein kinases and promotes neurite growth. J Biol Chem 2001;276(34): 31674–83.

[35] Li X, Bijur GN, Jope RS. Glycogen synthase kinase-3beta, mood stabilizers, and neuro-protection. Bipolar Disord 2002;4(2):137–44.

[36] Jorda EG, Verdaguer E, Morano A, et al. Lithium prevents colchicine-induced apoptosis in rat cerebellar granule neurons. Bipolar Disord 2004;6(2):144–9.

[37] Bijur GN, De Sarno P, Jope RS. Glycogen synthase kinase-3beta facilitates staurosporine- and heat shock-induced apoptosis. Protection by lithium. J Biol Chem 2000;275(11): 7583–90.

[38] Wei H, Leeds PR, Qian Y, et al. Beta-amyloid peptide-induced death of PC 12 cells and cerebellar granule cell neurons is inhibited by long-term lithium treatment. Eur J Pharmacol 2000;392(3):117–23.

[39] Peng G, Li G, Tzeng N, et al. Valproate pretreatment protects dopaminergic neurons from LPS-induced neurotoxicity in rat midbrain cultures: role of microglia. Brain Res Mol Brain Res, in press.

[40] Pardo R, Andreolotti AG, Ramos B, et al. Opposed effects of lithium on the MEK-ERK pathway in neural cells: inhibition in astrocytes and stimulation in neurons by GSK3 independent mechanisms. J Neurochem 2003;87(2):417–26.

[41] Song L, Zhou T, Jope RS. Lithium facilitates apoptotic signaling induced by activation of the Fas death domain-containing receptor. BMC Neurosci 2004;5(1):20.

[42] Hennion JP, el-Masri MA, Huff MO, et al. Evaluation of neuroprotection by lithium and valproic acid against ouabain-induced cell damage. Bipolar Disord 2002;4(3):201–6.

[43] Daniel ED, Mudge AW, Maycox PR. Comparative analysis of the effects of four mood stabilizers in SH-SY5Y cells and in primary neurons. Bipolar Disord 2005;7(1):33–41.

[44] Williams R, Ryves WJ, Dalton EC, et al. A molecular cell biology of lithium. Biochem Soc Trans 2004;32(Pt 5):799–802.

[45] Hashimoto R, Senatorov V, Kanai H, et al. Lithium stimulates progenitor proliferation in cultured brain neurons. Neuroscience 2003;117(1):55–61.

[46] Shimomura A, Nomura R, Senda T. Lithium inhibits apoptosis of mouse neural progenitor cells. Neuroreport 2003;14(14):1779–82.

[47] Laeng P, Pitts RL, Lemire AL, et al. The mood stabilizer valproic acid stimulates GABA neurogenesis from rat forebrain stem cells. J Neurochem 2004;91(1):238–51.

[48] Murray CJ, Lopez AD. Evidence-based health policy–lessons from the Global Burden of Disease Study. Science 1996;274(5288):740–3.

[49] Practice guideline for the treatment of patients with bipolar disorder (revision). Am J Psychiatry 2002;159(4 Suppl):1–50.

[50] Einat H, Manji HK, Belmaker RH. New approaches to modeling bipolar disorder. Psychopharmacol Bull 2003;37(1):47–63.

[51] Machado-Vieira R, Kapczinski F, Soares JC. Perspectives for the development of animal models of bipolar disorder. Prog Neuropsychopharmacol Biol Psychiatry 2004;28(2): 209–24.

[52] Nestler EJ, Barrot M, DiLeone RJ, et al. Neurobiology of depression. Neuron 2002;34(1): 13–25.

[53] Machado-Vieira R, Schmidt AP, Avila TT, et al. Increased cerebrospinal fluid levels of S100B protein in rat model of mania induced by ouabain. Life Sci 2004;76(7):805–11.

[54] el-Mallakh RS, Harrison LT, Li R, et al. An animal model for mania: preliminary results. Prog Neuropsychopharmacol Biol Psychiatry 1995;19(5):955–62.

[55] Li R, el-Mallakh RS, Harrison L, Changaris DG, et al. Lithium prevents ouabain-induced behavioral changes. Toward an animal model for manic depression. Mol Chem Neuropathol 1997;31(1):65–72.

[56] Wei Q, Lu XY, Liu L, et al. Glucocorticoid receptor overexpression in forebrain: a mouse model of increased emotional lability. Proc Natl Acad Sci U S A 2004;101(32): 11851–6.

[57] Ikonomov OC, Petrov T, Soden K, et al. Lithium treatment in ovo: effects on embryonic heart rate, natural death of ciliary ganglion neurons, and brain expression of a highly conserved chicken homolog of human MTG8/ETO. Brain Res Dev Brain Res 2000;123(1): 13–24.

[58] Cui SS, Yang CP, Bowen RC, et al. Valproic acid enhances axonal regeneration and recovery of motor function after sciatic nerve axotomy in adult rats. Brain Res 2003; 975(1–2):229–36.

[59] Youdim MB, Arraf Z. Prevention of MPTP (N-methyl-4-phenyl-1,2,3,6-tetrahydro-pyridine) dopaminergic neurotoxicity in mice by chronic lithium: involvements of Bcl-2 and Bax. Neuropharmacology 2004;46(8):1130–40.

[60] Ghribi O, Herman MM, Savory J. Lithium inhibits Abeta-induced stress in endoplasmic reticulum of rabbit hippocampus but does not prevent oxidative damage and tau phosphorylation. J Neurosci Res 2003;71(6):853–62.

[61] Wei H, Qin ZH, Senatorov VV, et al. Lithium suppresses excitotoxicity-induced striatal lesions in a rat model of Huntington's disease. Neuroscience 2001;106(3):603–12.

[62] Edmonds HL Jr, Jiang YD, Zhang PY, et al. Topiramate as a neuroprotectant in a rat model of global ischemia-induced neurodegeneration. Life Sci 2001;69(19):2265–77.

[63] Nonaka S, Chuang DM. Neuroprotective effects of chronic lithium on focal cerebral ischemia in rats. Neuroreport 1998;9(9):2081–4.

[64] Xu J, Culman J, Blume A, et al. Chronic treatment with a low dose of lithium protects the brain against ischemic injury by reducing apoptotic death. Stroke 2003;34(5):1287–92.

[65] Ren M, Senatorov VV, Chen RW, et al. Postinsult treatment with lithium reduces brain damage and facilitates neurological recovery in a rat ischemia/reperfusion model. Proc Natl Acad Sci U S A 2003;100(10):6210–5.

[66] Ma J, Zhang GY, Liu Y, et al. Lithium suppressed Tyr-402 phosphorylation of proline-rich tyrosine kinase (Pyk2) and interactions of Pyk2 and PSD-95 with NR2A in rat hippocampus following cerebral ischemia. Neurosci Res 2004;49(4):357–62.

[67] Son H, Yu IT, Hwang SJ, et al. Lithium enhances long-term potentiation independently of hippocampal neurogenesis in the rat dentate gyrus. J Neurochem 2003;85(4):872–81.

[68] Malberg JE, Eisch AJ, Nestler EJ, et al. Chronic antidepressant treatment increases neurogenesis in adult rat hippocampus. J Neurosci 2000;20(24):9104–10.

[69] Yu IT, Kim JS, Lee SH, et al. Chronic lithium enhances hippocampal long-term potentiation, but not neurogenesis, in the aged rat dentate gyrus. Biochem Biophys Res Commun 2003;303(4):1193–8.

[70] Sairanen M, Lucas G, Ernfors P, et al. Brain-derived neurotrophic factor and anti-depressant drugs have different but coordinated effects on neuronal turnover, proliferation, and survival in the adult dentate gyrus. J Neurosci 2005;25(5):1089–94.

[71] Santarelli L, Saxe M, Gross C, et al. Requirement of hippocampal neurogenesis for the behavioral effects of antidepressants. Science 2003;301(5634):805–9.

[72] Malberg JE, Duman RS. Cell proliferation in adult hippocampus is decreased by inescapable stress: reversal by fluoxetine treatment. Neuropsychopharmacology 2003; 28(9):1562–71.

[73] Vollmayr B, Simonis C, Weber S, et al. Reduced cell proliferation in the dentate gyrus is not correlated with the development of learned helplessness. Biol Psychiatry 2003;54(10): 1035–40.

[74] Scharfman HE. Functional implications of seizure-induced neurogenesis. Adv Exp Med Biol 2004;548:192–212.

[75] Haldane M, Frangou S. New insights help define the pathophysiology of bipolar affective disorder: neuroimaging and neuropathology findings. Prog Neuropsychopharmacol Biol Psychiatry 2004;28(6):943–60.

[76] Beyer JL, Krishnan KR. Volumetric brain imaging findings in mood disorders. Bipolar Disord 2002;4(2):89–104.

[77] Moore GJ, Bebchuk JM, Wilds IB, et al. Lithium-induced increase in human brain grey matter. Lancet 2000;356(9237):1241–2.

[78] Kieseppa T, van Erp TG, Haukka J, et al. Reduced left hemispheric white matter volume in twins with bipolar I disorder. Biol Psychiatry 2003;54(9):896–905.

[79] Sassi RB, Brambilla P, Hatch JP, et al. Reduced left anterior cingulate volumes in untreated bipolar patients. Biol Psychiatry 2004;56(7):467–75.

[80] Schlaepfer TE, Harris GJ, Tien AY, et al. Decreased regional cortical gray matter volume in schizophrenia. Am J Psychiatry 1994;151(6):842–8.

[81] Zipursky RB, Seeman MV, Bury A, et al. Deficits in gray matter volume are present in schizophrenia but not bipolar disorder. Schizophr Res 1997;26(2–3):85–92.

[82] Strakowski SM, Wilson DR, Tohen M, et al. Structural brain abnormalities in first-episode mania. Biol Psychiatry 1993;33(8–9):602–9.

[83] Harvey I, Persaud R, Ron MA, et al. Volumetric MRI measurements in bipolars compared with schizophrenics and healthy controls. Psychol Med 1994;24(3):689–99.

[84] Dupont RM, Jernigan TL, Heindel W, et al. Magnetic resonance imaging and mood disorders. Localization of white matter and other subcortical abnormalities. Arch Gen Psychiatry 1995;52(9):747–55.

[85] Pearlson GD, Barta PE, Powers RE, et al. Ziskind-Somerfeld Research Award 1996. Medial and superior temporal gyral volumes and cerebral asymmetry in schizophrenia versus bipolar disorder. Biol Psychiatry 1997;41(1):1–14.

[86] Brambilla P, Harenski K, Nicoletti M, et al. Differential effects of age on brain gray matter in bipolar patients and healthy individuals. Neuropsychobiology 2001;43(4):242–7.

[87] Lopez-Larson MP, DelBello MP, Zimmerman ME, et al. Regional prefrontal gray and white matter abnormalities in bipolar disorder. Biol Psychiatry 2002;52(2):93–100.

[88] Davis KA, Kwon A, Cardenas VA, et al. Decreased cortical gray and cerebral white matter in male patients with familial bipolar I disorder. J Affect Disord 2004;82(3):475–85.

[89] Lim KO, Rosenbloom MJ, Faustman WO, et al. Cortical gray matter deficit in patients with bipolar disorder. Schizophr Res 1999;40(3):219–27.

[90] Doris A, Belton E, Ebmeier KP, et al. Reduction of cingulate gray matter density in poor outcome bipolar illness. Psychiatry Res 2004;130(2):153–9.

[91] Strakowski SM, DelBello MP, Sax KW, et al. Brain magnetic resonance imaging of structural abnormalities in bipolar disorder. Arch Gen Psychiatry 1999;56(3):254–60.

[92] Drevets WC, Price JL, Simpson JR Jr, et al. Subgenual prefrontal cortex abnormalities in mood disorders. Nature 1997;386(6627):824–7.

[93] Hirayasu Y, Shenton ME, Salisbury DF, et al. Subgenual cingulate cortex volume in first-episode psychosis. Am J Psychiatry 1999;156(7):1091–3.

[94] Frangou S, Hadjulis M, Chitnis X, et al. The Maudsley Bipolar Disorder Project: brain structural changes in bipolar I disorder. Bipolar Disord 2002;4:123–4.

[95] Ongur D, Drevets WC, Price JL. Glial reduction in the subgenual prefrontal cortex in mood disorders. Proc Natl Acad Sci U S A 1998;95(22):13290–5.

[96] Rajkowska G, Halaris A, Selemon LD. Reductions in neuronal and glial density characterize the dorsolateral prefrontal cortex in bipolar disorder. Biol Psychiatry 2001;49(9):741–52.

[97] Benes FM, Vincent SL, Todtenkopf M. The density of pyramidal and nonpyramidal neurons in anterior cingulate cortex of schizophrenic and bipolar subjects. Biol Psychiatry 2001;50(6):395–406.

[98] Benes FM, Kwok EW, Vincent SL, et al. A reduction of nonpyramidal cells in sector CA2 of schizophrenics and manic depressives. Biol Psychiatry 1998;44(2):88–97.

[99] Baumann B, Danos P, Krell D, et al. Unipolar-bipolar dichotomy of mood disorders is supported by noradrenergic brainstem system morphology. J Affect Disord 1999;54(1–2): 217–24.

[100] Bowley MP, Drevets WC, Ongur D, et al. Low glial numbers in the amygdala in major depressive disorder. Biol Psychiatry 2002;52:404–12.

[101] Bowden CL. Making optimal use of combination pharmacotherapy in bipolar disorder. J Clin Psychiatry 2004;65(Suppl 15):21–4.

[102] Lingam R, Scott J. Treatment non-adherence in affective disorders. Acta Psychiatr Scand 2002;105(3):164–72.

ELSEVIER
SAUNDERS

Psychiatr Clin N Am
28 (2005) 415–425

PSYCHIATRIC
CLINICS
OF NORTH AMERICA

Bipolar Disorder and Substance Abuse

E. Sherwood Brown, MD, PhD

Psychoneuroendocrine Research Program, Department of Psychiatry,
University of Texas Southwestern Medical Center at Dallas, 5323 Harry Hines Boulevard,
Dallas, TX 75390, USA

Bipolar disorder (BPD) is a common, severe, and persistent psychiatric illness affecting 1.3% to 1.7% of the population [1,2]. Substance use disorders (SUDs) are also common. A community-based study found a lifetime prevalence of 17% for alcohol abuse or dependence and 6% for other substances [1]. BPD and SUDs occur together more frequently than would be expected by chance alone. This article discusses the prevalence of SUDs in patients with BPD, the impact of substance abuse on the treatment of BPD, possible reasons for the strong association between the two illnesses, and potential treatments. The topic of BPD and SUDs has been the subject of several reviews in the past several years focusing on various aspects of these disorders [3–6]. This article does not attempt to provide a comprehensive review of the topic but updates the information in previous reviews by discussing more recently published data and findings from some recent clinical trials.

Prevalence of substance use disorders in persons with bipolar disorder

Kessler [7] has recently reviewed the epidemiology of dual-diagnosis disorders. Three population-based studies have examined the prevalence of SUDs in persons with BPD [1,8,9]. Regier et al [1] used the National Institute of Mental Health Diagnostic Interview Schedule to assess psychiatric disorders in 20,291 respondents and found a 61% lifetime prevalence of SUDs in persons with bipolar I disorder and a 48% lifetime prevalence in those with bipolar II disorder, compared with 27% for persons with major depressive disorder, 47% for persons with schizophrenia, and 17% in the entire community sample. Although the prevalence of alcohol abuse and dependence in people with BPD (46%) seems to be higher than for all other

---

E-mail address: sherwood.brown@utsouthwestern.edu

0193-953X/05/$ - see front matter © 2005 Elsevier Inc. All rights reserved.
doi:10.1016/j.psc.2005.01.004

drugs combined (41%), the relative risk in BPD, compared with the general population, is greater for drugs for than alcohol-related disorders (odds ratios 11 versus 6).

Kessler et al [9] used the Composite International Diagnostic Interview to assess psychiatric disorders in 8098 respondents in the community. They found lifetime odds ratios in persons with a history of mania of 0.3 for alcohol abuse, 9.7 for alcohol dependence, 1.2 for drug abuse, 8.4 for drug dependence, and 6.8 for any SUD. In addition, Kessler et al found that most patients with affective disorders reported mood symptoms beginning either concurrently with or before the SUD.

In a recently published report, Grant et al [8] used the National Institute on Alcohol Abuse and Alcoholism Alcohol Use Disorder and Associated Disabilities Interview Schedule (*Diagnostic and Statistical Manual*-IV version) to assess illnesses in 43,093 respondents. Among all respondents, they found a 12-month prevalence of 1.7% for mania and of 1.2% for hypomania, percentages that remained virtually unchanged when persons with substance-induced mania or hypomania were excluded. In respondents with a 12-month history of an SUD, the prevalence of mania increased to 4.9% and hypomania to 3.3%. The 12-month prevalence of any SUD was 27.9% in those with a history of mania, 26.6% in those with hypomania, and 19.2% in those with major depressive disorder. Among respondents with BPD, the odds were higher for drug or alcohol dependence than for drug or alcohol abuse and were higher for those with a history of mania than for those with hypomania. For example, the odds ratio of drug abuse was 3.7 for persons with mania and 1.7 for persons with hypomania, whereas the odds ratio for drug dependence was 13.9 for persons with mania and 4.4 for persons with hypomania.

These data from community-based studies suggest that drug and alcohol abuse and dependence are much more common in persons with BPD than in the general population and are higher than for major depressive disorder and perhaps schizophrenia. Thus, the comorbidity between BPD and SUDs is strong. BPD seems to be associated with substance dependence more strongly than with abuse, suggesting that, when present, SUDs tend to be severe and disabling. Although alcohol-related disorders are more common in BPD and the general population than drug-related disorders, patients with BPD have a greater relative risk compared to the general population, of developing a drug-related disorder than an alcohol-related disorder. Thus, a person with BPD is more likely to develop an alcohol-related disorder than a drug-related disorder, but is at greater relative risk than the general population of developing a drug-related disorder than an alcohol-related disorder. The findings by Kessler et al [9] that most respondents developed BPD before developing substance use and the finding by Grant et al [8] that few respondents seemed to have substance-induced mood disorders suggest that the association between BPD and substance abuse is probably not, in most cases, secondary to the mood effects of the substances.

One topic not addressed by the large, community-based studies is the specific drugs abused by persons with BPD. No studies with large sample sizes have addressed this question. A small study by Estroff et al [10] examined this question in a clinical sample, using structured interviews in a group of 36 inpatients with BPD, and found lifetime rates of SUDs of 64% for cannabis, 39% for cocaine, 39% for amphetamines, 31% for hallucinogens, 25% for opiates, and 11% for phencyclidine.

Risk factors for substance use disorders in persons with bipolar disorder

Sonne et al [11] identified male gender, lower education, and the presence of other Axis I illnesses as risk factors for drug abuse in patients with BPD. Thus, male gender, a risk factor for an SUD in the general population, seems to be associated with SUDs in patients with BPD. The findings also suggest that an additional psychiatric comorbidity may have an additive effect on the risk of SUD. Anxiety disorders and other illnesses are common in patients with BPD [12], and the presence of these other psychiatric illnesses could contribute to the increased prevalence of substance abuse in this population.

One study that included BPD participants looked at the association between anxiety disorders and SUDs among patients with severe affective disorders (N = 260) [13]. In the BPD patients in the study (n = 33), the odds ratio for cocaine use disorder with anxiety disorder was 4.2, whereas the odds ratio for alcohol use disorder with anxiety disorder was 1.3. These findings suggest that anxiety disorders are associated with SUDs in patients with BPD, and that cocaine-use disorders are more strongly associated with anxiety disorders than are alcohol-use disorders.

Another factor that affects substance use patterns is mood state. In patients with BPD, mood can fluctuate between depression, mania, mixed states, and euthymia. The type or amount of substances used could fluctuate as mood state changes. The role of mood state as a risk factor for drug abuse has been examined in several investigations. Estroff et al [10] reported a trend toward greater polysubstance and amphetamine abuse of drugs during mania than during depression. Sonne et al [11] reported more alcohol use during the manic phase but more cocaine use during the depressed phase.

In studies by the authors' group examining persons with BPD and SUDs during clinical trials, stronger positive associations were found between changes in cocaine use or craving and changes in depressive symptoms than changes in manic symptoms [14,15]. In contrast, changes in alcohol-related outcomes were more strongly associated with changes in manic symptoms rather than depressive symptoms (Brown, unpublished data). The cause and effect cannot be determined, but the findings might suggest that people with BPD use more cocaine when depressed and use more alcohol when manic.

Strakowski et al [16] examined associations between alcohol and cannabis use in a group of 50 patients with BPD followed for up to 24 months. They found that duration of alcohol use was associated with time depressed, whereas duration of cannabis use was associated with time in a manic state. Some reports also suggest that mixed or dysphoric mania, characterized by manic and depressive symptoms occurring at the same time, may be more strongly associated with substance use than is pure or euphoric mania [11,17–19].

Impact of a substance use disorder on bipolar depression

The presence of an SUD seems to have a negative impact on the course of BPD. Several studies report increased hospitalization in BPD patients with an SUD [11,20–24]. Cassidy et al [24] examined 392 patients hospitalized for manic or mixed episodes, finding that a lifetime history of an SUD was associated with significantly more lifetime hospitalizations. The results are somewhat mixed, however, with other studies not finding an association between drug abuse and severity of psychopathology, rate or length of hospitalization, or mental health service utilization [25–27]. Mueser et al [28] even reported significantly fewer prior hospitalizations in bipolar persons with cocaine abuse.

In patients with BPD, a SUD seems to be associated with increased risk of violence toward self and others. Potash et al [29] reported that 38% of a sample of patients with SUDs and alcohol dependence had a lifetime suicide attempt compared to 22% of those with BPD but no alcohol dependence. In addition, they found a clustering of BPD, alcohol dependence, and suicide attempts in some families, potentially consistent with inheritance of genetic traits that might lead to these features. In another study, aggression and violence were significantly greater in psychotic patients with comorbid drug abuse, a subset of whom had bipolar and schizoaffective disorders, than in the control group [30]. Comtois et al [31] recently examined a group of 7819 inpatients with BPD, major depressive disorder, schizoaffective disorder, or schizophrenia and found that current SUDs were associated with lifetime suicide attempts, suicidal ideation, or recent attempts at hospital admission.

The presence of an SUD seems to be associated with poor treatment adherence in patients with BPD. Keck et al [32] followed 134 patients with BPD for up to 12 months after a hospitalization for a manic or mixed episode. The only characteristic that was associated with treatment non-adherence was the presence of an SUD. In those with an SUD, only 32% were fully adherent with treatment compared to 58% in those without an SUD. Similarly, Goldberg et al [33], in a retrospective analysis of 204 inpatients with bipolar I disorder, found that 53% of those with substance abuse had a history of medication nonadherence compared with only 35% among those without substance abuse.

Adherence with lithium may be especially poor in patients with both BPD and an SUD. Aagaard and Vestergaard [34] found a significant association between drug abuse and nonadherence with lithium therapy in a group of patients with affective disorders. Weiss et al [35] reported greater adherence with valproate than lithium in BPD patients with SUDs.

Given the association of substance use with treatment nonadherence, poor response to mood stabilizers, violence, and hospitalization, one might predict that patients with BPD and SUDs would have a poor response to substance abuse treatment. This topic has had little research. Findings from one study suggest that persons with BPD in substance abuse treatment showed a trend toward greater drug use before and during treatment, more frequent suicidal thoughts, and more episodes of violence than subjects without affective illness [36]. Thus, SUDs may lead to a poor BPD prognosis, and BPD may be associated with a poor response to substance abuse treatment.

Mixed results are reported as to whether persons with an SUD and BPD have an earlier onset of mood symptoms than those without an SUD. Winokur et al [37] reported an earlier onset of affective symptoms in BPD patients with an SUD. Strakowski et al [38] found no association between drug abuse and age of onset of mood symptoms but a significantly later onset of affective illness with alcohol abuse.

Causes of substance abuse disorders in patients with bipolar disorder

Several previous reviews have addressed aspects of the strong association between BPD and substance use disorder [4,6,39]. At least three possible explanations can be postulated: (1) BPD causes SUDs; (2) SUDs cause BPD; and (3) BPD and SUDs share some common origin. The idea that BPD causes SUDs would suggest that BPD should occur before the SUD. The literature suggests that this priority occurs in approximately half of all patients. Because both disorders frequently have their onset in adolescence or young adulthood, and because determining the onset of BPD symptoms can be challenging, it is difficult in many cases to determine which came first. If BPD causes SUDs, then one could predict that amelioration of mood symptoms would effectively treat the substance abuse. The data are mixed in this regard, with some studies suggesting persons with SUDS abuse substances in all mood states and other suggesting a relationship between substance use and mood state. BPD could also lead to substance use secondary to psychosocial changes from the illness. For example, BPD could result in homelessness or living in shelters and boarding homes, leading to in greater exposure to substance use and increased vulnerability to developing an SUD.

If SUDs cause BPD, one would predict an onset of substance use before the onset of mood symptoms. This priority seems to occur in many, but clearly not all, patients with both disorders [4]. Thus, this possibility does not explain the substantial number of cases in which the mood disorder occurs first. Substance use could lead to symptoms secondary to the substances that are similar to those of BPD. As the author and colleagues [3] discussed in an earlier review, misdiagnosis may explain some of the bipolar spectrum disorders diagnosed in persons in substance abuse treatment settings. If one assumes that the full syndrome of mania is less likely than milder hypomania to result from substance use, misdiagnosis would not seem to explain the high prevalence of SUDs found in community samples of persons with bipolar I disorder. In addition, in the most recent comorbidity study, Grant et al [8] carefully excluded likely cases of substance-induced mood disorders and still found a high prevalence of SUDs in persons with BPD.

Finally, the two disorders could share a common origin. Both BPD and SUD seem to be in part caused by genetic vulnerability. Genetic similarities of the two disorders have not been thoroughly investigated, but data from studies of first-degree relatives of persons with BPD, which find elevated rates of BPD but not SUDs, do not seem to support this idea [4]. In addition, features of BPD (eg, impulsivity) that remain even after effective treatment of the mood symptoms are also features of substance-related disorder and could explain their frequent co-occurrence.

Treatment of patients with bipolar disorder and a substance use disorder

In a recent review, Kosten and Kosten [40] proposed that the ideal medication for the treatment of BPD and SUDs would be effective in treating BPD symptoms, reduce withdrawal or craving, prevent relapse after the withdrawal period, have minimal abuse potential, require infrequent dosing, and have a favorable side-effect profile. Although no currently available medication meets all these criteria, promising results have been reported with medications that meet some of these criteria. Persons with SUDs frequently are excluded from clinical trials of patients with BPD, but treatment research in dual-diagnosis patients seems to have increased in recent years.

To date, four randomized, placebo-controlled trials and one randomized, open-label, controlled trial have been conducted in persons with BPD and an SUD (Table 1). Geller et al [41] examined lithium versus placebo in 25 adolescent patients with bipolar I disorder, bipolar II disorder, or recurrent major depressive disorder and comorbid substance abuse (primarily of alcohol and marijuana). During 6 weeks of follow-up, participants taking lithium had a significant decrease in the number of positive urine drug screens ($P = 0.042$).

Brady et al [42] reported greater reduction in cocaine-positive urine screens and depressive symptom severity with carbamazepine than with

Table 1
Controlled medication trials that included patients with bipolar disorder and a substance use disorder

Author	Medication	Sample	Design	Findings
Geller et al [41]	Lithium	25 adolescents with affective and substance use disorders	6-week randomized double-blind placebo-controlled	Fewer positive urine drug screens in lithium group
Brady et al [42]	Carbamazepine	57 adults with affective disorder and cocaine dependence	12-week randomized double-blind placebo-controlled	Decreased cocaine use with carbamazepine compared with placebo
Salloum et al [43]	Valproate	52 adults with bipolar I disorder and alcohol dependence	24-week randomized double-blind placebo-controlled	Less alcohol use in valproate group
Brown et al [4]	Quetiapine	29 adults with psychiatric illness and stimulant-related disorder receiving neuroleptic agents	12-week randomized open-label switch to quetiapine versus treatment as usual	Improvement in psychiatric symptoms and decreased drug craving in quetiapine group

placebo in cocaine-dependent patients with mood disorders (major depressive disorder or BPD) (n = 57) but not in a group of patients with cocaine dependence without mood disorders (n = 82).

Salloum et al [43] randomly assigned 52 outpatients with bipolar I disorder and alcohol dependence for 24 weeks of treatment with valproate plus treatment as usual or placebo plus treatment as usual. The valproate group had significantly fewer heavy drinking days and a trend toward fewer drinks per heavy drinking day than the placebo group. The two groups had similar improvement in manic and depressive symptomatology, suggesting that the reduction in alcohol consumption was not caused primarily by improvement in mood.

The authors' group randomly assigned 29 outpatients with major mental illness and stimulant abuse/dependence who were receiving traditional neuroleptic agents (13 had bipolar I disorder) either to continue therapy with the neuroleptic or to switch to open-label quetiapine using an overlap and taper method [44]. Significant improvement in psychiatric symptoms and drug craving were found in the group switched to quetiapine compared with the neuroleptic group.

Several uncontrolled trials in patients with BPD and an SUD have been recently published. The authors' group [14] reported positive results with open-label quetiapine add-on therapy in 17 patients with BPD and cocaine dependence. Significant improvement in psychiatric symptoms and cocaine craving and trends toward decreases in cocaine use were found. Participants in this study who had alcohol-related disorders in addition to the cocaine dependence showed a reduction in alcohol craving and use with quetiapine [45]. In another study by the author's group [46], 20 antipsychotic-treated patients with BPD or schizoaffective disorder and current SUD were switched to open-label aripiprazole using an overlap and taper method. Significant improvements in manic and depressive symptoms were observed. Cocaine and alcohol craving was also reduced.

A better understanding of the causes of SUDs in people with BPD might better inform treatment research. If SUDs are primarily a result of the symptoms of BPD, medications that are effective for mood symptoms and psychotic features should also decrease substance use. Medications that are ineffective in pure substance abuse might be effective for substance abuse in BPD, as Brady et al [42] found with carbamazepine. As discussed previously, substance use in BPD seems to be related in part to mood symptoms. Thus, lithium, anticonvulsants, and antipsychotic agents are potential treatments. When substance use is unrelated to the presence of BPD symptoms, however, treatment might focus on medications that specifically target substance use. Trials of currently available medications for SUDs such as naltrexone, acamprosate, and buprenorphine are needed. In addition, given the promising results reported with topiramate in people with pure alcohol dependence [47], trials in people with BPD and alcohol dependence seem warranted.

Psychotherapeutic approaches have also been explored for BPD and SUD [48]. Two cognitive behavioral therapy approaches have been developed specifically for persons with BPD and an SUD. Schmitz et al [49] have developed a manual-driven cognitive behavioral therapy approach specifically designed for persons with BPD and substance abuse [49]. The investigators randomly assigned 46 patients with BPD and SUD to the intervention plus medication monitoring or to medication monitoring alone for 12 weeks. They found that persons receiving the therapy remained in treatment longer than those not receiving cognitive behavioral therapy and had better medication adherence and improvement in mood but did not show greater improvement in substance-related outcomes.

Weiss et al [50] have developed a manual-driven, cognitive behavioral–based relapse-prevention treatment called Integrated Group Therapy that focuses on both BPD and substance use. This approach was examined in 45 persons with BPD and SUD using a 6-month, nonrandomized design. Results suggested greater abstinence from substances in the group receiving the intervention (n = 21) than in controls (n = 24).

Summary

SUDs are common in people with BPD. The reasons for this association are not well understood and may be related to several factors. When present, SUDs in BPD patients seem to be associated with a poor prognosis. The treatment of patients with BPD and an SUD has been the subject of relatively little investigation, but medications that are effective mood stabilizers seem to decrease substance use in some reports.

References

[1] Regier DA, Farmer ME, Rae DS, et al. Comorbidity of mental disorders with alcohol and other drug abuse. JAMA 1990;264:2511–8.

[2] Kessler RC, McGonagle KA, Zhao S, et al. Lifetime and 12-month prevalence of DSM-III-R psychiatric disorders in the United States. Results from the National Comorbidity Survey. Arch Gen Psychiatry 1994;51:8–19.

[3] Brown ES, Suppes T, Adinoff B, et al. Drug abuse and bipolar disorder: comorbidity or misdiagnosis? J Affect Disord 2001;65:105–15.

[4] Strakowski SM, DelBello MP. The co-occurrence of bipolar and substance use disorders. Clin Psychol Rev 2000;20:191–206.

[5] Albanese MJ, Pies R. The bipolar patient with comorbid substance use disorder: recognition and management. CNS Drugs 2004;18:585–96.

[6] Levin FR, Hennessy G. Bipolar disorder and substance abuse. Biol Psychiatry 2004;56: 738–48.

[7] Kessler RC. The epidemiology of dual diagnosis. Biol Psychiatry 2004;56(10):730–7.

[8] Grant BF, Stinson FS, Dawson DA, et al. Prevalence and co-occurrence of substance use disorders and independent mood and anxiety disorders: results from the National Epidemiologic Survey on Alcohol and Related Conditions. Arch Gen Psychiatry 2004;61: 807–16.

[9] Kessler RC, Nelson CB, McGonagle KA, et al. The epidemiology of co-occurring addictive and mental disorders: implications for prevention and service utilization. Am J Orthopsychiatry 1996;66:17–31.

[10] Estroff TW, Dackis CA, Gold MS, et al. Drug abuse and bipolar disorders. Int J Psychiatry Med 1985;15:37–40.

[11] Sonne SC, Brady KT, Morton WA. Substance abuse and bipolar affective disorder. J Nerv Ment Dis 1994;182:349–52.

[12] Perugi G, Toni C, Akiskal HS. Anxious-bipolar comorbidity. Diagnostic and treatment challenges. Psychiatr Clin North Am 1999;22:565–83 [viii.].

[13] Goodwin RD, Stayner DA, Chinman MJ, et al. The relationship between anxiety and substance use disorders among individuals with severe affective disorders. Compr Psychiatry 2002;43:245–52.

[14] Brown ES, Nejtek VA, Perantie DC, et al. Quetiapine in bipolar disorder and cocaine dependence. Bipolar Disord 2002;4:406–11.

[15] Brown ES, Nejtek VA, Perantie DC, et al. Lamotrigine in patients with bipolar disorder and cocaine dependence. J Clin Psychiatry 2003;64:197–201.

[16] Strakowski SM, DelBello MP, Fleck DE, et al. The impact of substance abuse on the course of bipolar disorder. Biol Psychiatry 2000;48:477–85.

[17] Himmelhoch JM, Mulla D, Neil JF, et al. Incidence and significance of mixed affective states in a bipolar population. Arch Gen Psychiatry 1976;33:1062–6.

[18] McElroy SL, Keck PE Jr, Pope HG Jr, et al. Hypothalamic-pituitary-adrenocortical function in mixed and pure mania. Acta Psychiatr Scand 1992;85:270–4.

[19] Feinman JA, Dunner DL. The effect of alcohol and substance abuse on the course of bipolar affective disorder. J Affect Disord 1996;37:43–9.

[20] Haywood TW, Karvitz HM, Grossman LS, et al. Predicting the "revolving door" phenomenon among patients with schizophrenic, schizoaffective, and affective disorders. Am J Psychiatry 1995;152:856–61.

[21] Himmelhoch JM, Garfinkel M. Sources of lithium resistance in mixed mania. Psychopharmacol Bull 1986;22:613–20.

[22] O'Connell R, Mayo J, Flatow L, et al. Outcome of bipolar disorder on long-term treatment with lithium. Br J Psychiatry 1991;159:123–9.

[23] Tohen M, Waternaux C, Tsuang M. Outcome in mania, a 4-year prospective follow-up of 75 patients utilizing survival analysis. Arch Gen Psychiatry 1990;47:1106–11.

[24] Cassidy F, Ahearn EP, Carroll BJ. Substance abuse in bipolar disorder. Bipolar Disord 2001;3:181–8.

[25] Bauer MS, Shea N, McBride L, et al. Predictors of service utilization in veterans with bipolar disorder: a prospective study. J Affect Disord 1997;44:159–68.

[26] Bradley CJ, Zarkin GA. Inpatient stays for patients diagnosed with severe psychiatric disorders and substance abuse. Health Serv Res 1996;31:339–408.

[27] Warner R, Taylor D, Wright J, et al. Substance use among the mentally ill: prevalence, reasons for use, and effects on illness. Am J Orthopsychiatry 1994;64:30–9.

[28] Mueser KT, Yarnold PR, Bellack AS. Diagnostic and demographic correlates of substance abuse in schizophrenia and major affective disorder. Acta Psychiatr Scand 1992;85:48–55.

[29] Potash JB, Kane HS, Chiu YF, et al. Attempted suicide and alcoholism in bipolar disorder: clinical and familial relationships. Am J Psychiatry 2000;157:2048–50.

[30] Scott H, Johnson S, Menezes P, et al. Substance misuse and risk of aggression and offending among the severely mentally ill. Br J Psychiatry 1998;172:345–50.

[31] Comtois KA, Russo JE, Roy-Byrne P, et al. Clinicians' assessments of bipolar disorder and substance abuse as predictors of suicidal behavior in acutely hospitalized psychiatric inpatients. Biol Psychiatry 2004;56:757–63.

[32] Keck PE Jr, McElroy SL, Strakowski SM, et al. 12-month outcome of patients with bipolar disorder following hospitalization for a manic or mixed episode. Am J Psychiatry 1998;155: 646–52.

[33] Goldberg JF, Garno JL, Leon AC, et al. A history of substance abuse complicates remission from acute mania in bipolar disorder. J Clin Psychiatry 1999;60:733–40.

[34] Aagaard J, Vestergaard P. Predictors of outcome in prophylactic lithium treatment: a 2-year prospective study. J Affect Disord 1989;12:259–66.

[35] Weiss RD, Greenfield SF, Najavits LM, et al. Medication compliance among patients with bipolar disorder and substance use disorder. J Clin Psychiatry 1998;59:172–4.

[36] Saxon AJ, Calsyn DA, Stanton V, et al. Using the general behavior inventory to screen for mood disorders among patients with psychoactive substance dependence. Am J Addict 1994; 3:296–305.

[37] Winokur G, Turvey C, Akiskal H, et al. Alcoholism and drug abuse in three groups—bipolar I, unipolars and their acquaintances. J Affect Disord 1998;50:81–9.

[38] Strakowski SM, McElroy SL, Keck PE Jr, et al. The effects of antecedent substance abuse on the development of first-episode psychotic mania. J Psychiatr Res 1996;30:59–68.

[39] Swann AC. Manic-depressive illness and substance abuse. Psychiatr Ann 1997;27: 507–11.

[40] Kosten TR, Kosten TA. New medication strategies for comorbid substance use and bipolar affective disorders. Biol Psychiatry 2004;56:771–7.

[41] Geller B, Cooper TB, Sun K, et al. Double-blind and placebo-controlled study of lithium for adolescent bipolar disorders with secondary substance dependency. J Am Acad Child Adolesc Psychiatry 1998;37:171–8.

[42] Brady KT, Sonne SC, Malcolm RJ, et al. Carbamazepine in the treatment of cocaine dependence: subtyping by affective disorder. Exp Clin Psychopharmacol 2002;10:276–85.

[43] Salloum IM, Cornelius JR, Daley DC, et al. Efficacy of valproate maintenance in patients with bipolar disorder and alcoholism. A double-blind, placebo-controlled study. Arch Gen Psychiatry 2005;62:37–45.

[44] Brown ES, Nejtek VA, Perantie DC, et al. Cocaine and amphetamine use in patients with psychiatric illness: a randomized trial of typical antipsychotic continuation or discontinuation. J Clin Psychopharmacol 2003;23:384–8.

[45] Longoria J, Brown ES, Perantie DC, et al. Quetiapine for alcohol use and craving in bipolar disorder. J Clin Psychopharmacol 2004;24:101–2.

[46] Brown ES, Jeffress J, Liggin JDM, et al. Switching outpatients with bipolar or schizoaffective disorders and substance misuse from their current antipsychotic to aripiprazole. J Clin Psychiatry, in press.

[47] Johnson BA, Ait-Daoud N, Bowden CL, et al. Oral topiramate for treatment of alcohol dependence: a randomised controlled trial. Lancet 2003;361:1677–85.

[48] Carroll KM. Behavioral therapies for co-occurring substance use and mood disorders. Biol Psychiatry 2004;56:778–84.

[49] Schmitz JM, Averill P, Sayre S, et al. Cognitive-behavioral treatment of bipolar disorder and substance abuse: a preliminary randomized study. Addictive Disorders and Their Treatment 2002;1:17–24.

[50] Weiss RD, Griffin ML, Greenfield SF, et al. Group therapy for patients with bipolar disorder and substance dependence: results of a pilot study. J Clin Psychiatry 2000;61:361–7.

PSYCHIATRIC
CLINICS
OF NORTH AMERICA

Psychiatr Clin N Am
28 (2005) 427–441

ELSEVIER
SAUNDERS

Cognition in Bipolar Disorder

I. Julian Osuji, PhD[a], C. Munro Cullum, PhD[b],*

[a]Department of Psychiatry, The University of Texas Southwestern Medical Center at Dallas,
5323 Harry Hines Boulevard, Dallas, Dallas, TX 75390, USA
[b]Departments of Psychiatry and Neurology, The University of Texas
Southwestern Medical Center at Dallas, 5323 Harry Hines Boulevard,
Dallas, Dallas, TX 75390, USA

Bipolar disorder

According to the *Diagnostic and Statistical Manual of Mental Disorders–Fourth Edition*, bipolar I disorder is characterized by the occurrence of one or more manic or mixed episodes. One or more major depressive episodes are also common. Lifetime prevalence estimates for bipolar I disorder range from 0.4% to 1.6% [1]. Other subtypes include bipolar II disorder, characterized by one or more major depressive episodes accompanied by at least one hypomanic episode. Regardless of its label or subtype, the recurrent symptomatic nature of bipolar disorder (BPD) remains a consistent feature of this spectrum of illnesses.

BPD influences multiple aspects of behavior, which may affect daily functioning, including cognitive skills. It is difficult to estimate the prevalence of cognitive dysfunction in BPD, because the neuropsychologic presentation of the illness varies, and methodologic, clinical, and diagnostic differences across studies make direct comparisons difficult. Furthermore, even though the consensus is that BPD is associated with cognitive dysfunction, some individuals with BPD show no evidence of cognitive impairment. The level of cognitive impairment associated with BPD, when present, tends to be less severe than that seen in schizophrenia. As with schizophrenia, however, no single cognitive profile characterizes all patients with BPD, although some general trends and characteristics have been described. For instance, impulsivity, decreased inhibition, and distractibility characterize the manic episode, although various other cognitive state and trait

This work was supported in part by a grant from the National Institutes of Health; NIH T-32- MH067543-01.

* Corresponding author.
E-mail address: Munro.Cullum@UTSouthwestern.edu (C.M. Cullum).

symptoms have been reported. Attention/concentration or vigilance is often compromised in patients with BPD, whether experiencing acute depression or mania [2]. Difficulties with abstract thinking and problem solving, as well as with learning and memory, have been reported with some frequency. Deficits or disruptions in any of these or other aspects of cognition may affect daily functioning and have implications for diagnosis and treatment. Thus, from a clinical standpoint, the evaluation of cognitive abilities in patients with BPD is important. Neuropsychologic studies of BPD may also yield information useful in the understanding of the underlying cognitive and neuroanatomic systems involved.

What is neuropsychology?

Neuropsychology is a field dedicated to the study of brain–behavior relationships, and clinical neuropsychology is one of the applied sciences concerned with the assessment and treatment of brain dysfunction. Clinical neuropsychology is a recognized specialty within professional psychology and requires advanced training beyond traditional clinical psychology. Board certification in clinical neuropsychology is also possible through the American Board of Clinical Neuropsychology/American Board of Professional Psychology. Neuropsychologic or neuropsychometric tools are the tests and instruments designed to quantify cognitive functioning and to evaluate an individual's or group's specific strengths and weaknesses across a variety of cognitive domains. The neuropsychologic evaluation can be regarded as an expanded examination of mental status, which taps multiple cognitive skills and domains in a much more detailed and quantifiable fashion. Neuropsychologic techniques are recognized neurodiagnostic procedures [3] with their own Current Procedural Terminology (CPT) codes.

One role of the neuropsychologist is to sort out the factors that influence neurocognitive patterns of test results to understand disease expression, progression, or recovery. Neuropsychologists, along with other clinical and cognitive scientists, are also involved in research of brain–behavior relationships and use test results to improve the understanding of neuropsychiatric disorders, including the diagnosis, evaluation, care, and treatment of patients with known or suspected brain dysfunction.

The neuropsychologic evaluation

The neuropsychologic evaluation typically consists of a clinical interview, covering early development, educational and vocational history, neuro-medical risk factors, and other pertinent historical and current factors (eg, medication, mood state) that might influence cognitive performance. A central component of the neuropsychologic evaluation is the administration of standardized, objective tests of neurocognitive functioning. Hundreds of clinical and experimental neuropsychologic tests are available, although some enjoy more widespread use in clinical and clinical research settings.

The neuropsychologic evaluation operates on a model of assessing cognitive deficits and strengths by comparing individual test results with normative data and examining test scores in relation to each other within the context of an individual patient's background. Factors that may affect neuropsychologic test performance and interpretation include demographic variables such as age, education, gender, ethnicity, and socioeconomic status. Interpretation of test scores involves the integration of the statistical (data/results) and observational findings, history (medical records review and interview), and knowledge of the mechanisms of brain function and dysfunction to make sense of the person's cognitive functioning and clinical presentation.

When all these factors are considered together, the neuropsychologist looks for consistent patterns or cognitive profiles that tend to be seen in specific brain disorders [4]. In this way, test results can be used to assist in differential diagnosis of neuropsychiatric disorders and identification of comorbid processes, documenting impairments, understanding cognitive strengths and weaknesses, and tracking cognitive changes over time. Many standard clinical and experimental neuropsychologic or neurocognitive tests are available and often are combined into test "batteries". In the research setting, the choice of tests should be guided by the hypotheses of the investigation as they relate to cognitive functioning and by the nature of the disorder being studied. In clinical settings, the selection of examination procedures and tests should be guided by the patient's presenting complaints, referral questions, or diagnosis. Feedback of assessment results to the referral source and to the patient and the patient's family or caregiver typically includes overall impressions and recommendations and should highlight implications for the patient's everyday functioning.

Cognitive domains assessed

There are many ways to conceptualize and classify cognitive abilities, although some major rubrics are commonly used. These categories include global cognitive functioning, intellectual functioning, academic achievement, attention/concentration, executive function, language, visuospatial abilities, learning and memory, and psychomotor performance. Intellect or some estimate of general cognitive ability ("g"), which provides information useful in interpreting specific cognitive findings and an overall characterization of an individual's global cognitive status, is often assessed as part of a thorough neurocognitive examination. Individual cognitive domains are assessed by specialized pencil-paper, question-answer, or computerized tests, and some assessment of the patient's emotional status often completes the evaluation. Table 1 lists the primary cognitive domains assessed by a comprehensive neurocognitive evaluation and some common representative tests in each domain. For a more detailed listing and description of clinical and experimental neuropsychologic measures, the reader is referred to the excellent text by Lezak [5].

Table 1
Evaluating neurocognitive domains

Domains	Commonly used tests
Global cognition	MMSE, Mattis Dementia Rating Scale (DRS, DRS-2)
Intellectual functioning	Wechsler Adult Intelligence Scale-III, WASI, Shipley
Academic achievement	WRAT-3, PIAT-R, WJ-III; WIAT
Attention/concentration; mental tracking; processing speed	WAIS-III Digit Span, Continuous Performance Test, WAIS-III Digit Symbol, Symbol Digit Modalities Test, Trail Making Test, Stroop Test, Paced Auditory Serial Addition Test, Digit Vigilance Test, WAIS-III Letter-Number Sequencing
Executive functions, problem solving/concept formation, reasoning, cognitive flexibility	Wisconsin Card Sorting Test, Category Test, Trail Making B, Color Trails, Phonemic Fluency, Ruff Figural Fluency Test, Delis-Kaplan Executive Function System
Language	Boston Naming Test, WAIS-III Vocabulary; Verbal Fluency
Visuospatial	WAIS-III Block Design, Rey-Osterrieth Complex Figure, Clock Drawing Test, Judgment of Line Orientation
Learning and memory	California Verbal Learning Test (CVLT, CVLT-II), Wechsler Memory Scale-3rd edition (eg, Logical Memory, Visual Reproduction), Rey Auditory Verbal Learning Test, Hopkins Verbal Learning Test, Rey-Osterrieth Complex Figure Recall, Recognition Memory Test
Psychomotor	Finger Tapping Test, Grooved Pegboard, Grip Strength

Abbreviations: MMSE, Mini-Mental State Examination; PIAT-R, Peabody Individual Achievement Test Revised; WASI, Wechsler Abbreviated Scale of Intelligence; WIAT, Wechsler Individual Test of Achievement; WJ-III, Woodcock Johnson Tests of Cognition and Achievement; WRAT-3, Wide Range Achievement Test 3rd edition.

Orientation and level of arousal are important components of the neurobehavioral mental status examination and neurocognitive evaluation because assessment of other neurocognitive skills depends upon these basic building blocks of cognitive function. Depending upon the purpose of the evaluation and presenting symptoms, some neuropsychologic evaluations include a quantified assessment of simple and complex sensory skills (eg, simple touch, tactile discrimination, double-simultaneous stimulation, finger gnosis, graphesthesia) or motor skills (eg, grip strength, fine motor speed, dexterity, sequencing). Simple attention (eg, repeating digits forward) and sustained concentration or vigilance, as well as mental processing speed, are often examined. Other related tasks evaluate divided attention, mental manipulation/control and resistance to interference. Executive functioning refers to higher-order cognitive skills such as problem solving, reasoning, and mental flexibility and involves the integration and regulation of other cognitive abilities and behavioral responses. Language is assessed with respect to expressive abilities (eg, speaking, naming, writing, fluency) and receptive abilities (eg, comprehension, reading). Visuospatial abilities involve skills such as drawing, constructional skills, ability to perceive and reproduce geometric designs, and perceptual integration. Memory refers to a broad set of abilities and should not be regarded as a unitary phenomenon. Working memory, for example, is closely related to attention because it involves keeping a limited amount of information active and readily accessible for a brief period. Learning and memory are inextricably linked and involve the ability to encode, store, and retrieve information. In most clinical settings, episodic or declarative memory is assessed, which is the ability to learn and retrieve information presented at a particular point in time. This ability may be assessed through both visual and auditory modalities and generally requires learning and delayed recall of previously presented material (eg, word lists, stories, geometric designs). Last, many neuropsychologic evaluations include an assessment of mood or personality functioning, because such factors may relate to neurocognitive status, diagnosis, or outcome.

These cognitive domains and related functions and tests are indirect measures of various underlying brain systems, although most neurocognitive tests require multiple abilities, and hence many are not direct measures of focal cortical functioning. Table 2 presents a general overview of major brain divisions and some of their associated neurobehavioral and neurocognitive correlates.

Neurocognitive correlates of bipolar disorder

Many neuropsychiatric disorders are accompanied by cognitive symptoms, most notably schizophrenia, unipolar depression (UPD), and BPD. Although the extent of dysfunction varies depending upon the subtype, cognitive impairment is particularly common in schizophrenia-spectrum disorders. Patients with schizophrenia typically demonstrate a variety of cognitive deficits and reduced intellectual abilities, although this is not

Table 2
Neuropsychological functions by lobe*

Frontal	Temporal	Parietal	Occipital
Simple motor dexterity	Receptive language	Tactile sensation	Vision
Expressive language	Episodic memory	Stereognosis	Visual perception and
Verbal fluency	(verbal + nonverbal)	Graphesthesia	association
Executive functions	Emotional function	Visuospatial function	
Working memory	Receptive prosody	Praxis	
Complex reasoning		Reading	
and abstraction		Calculation	
Attention/processing		Visual Gestalt	
speed		processing	
Expressive prosody			

* This table is presented as a general categorization schema. Various functions are assessed by cognitive tests, which may tap several areas and may not specifically localize.

universally the case. Often these patients show pronounced problems in executive functioning and verbal learning and memory, although no specific pattern of cognitive deficits characterizes this heterogeneous group [6,7]. Neurocognitive variables have also proven to be significant predictors of a variety of outcome factors including daily functioning [8].

Neuropsychologic deficits related to UPD have also been reported, along with functional neuroimaging results, suggesting dysfunction of cortical-limbic circuits [9,10]. The most widely accepted finding with regard to the neuropsychology of depression is that cognitive impairment, when present, typically includes problems with attention and concentration, learning, and, in some cases, executive function [11]. Some of these symptoms may be transient and state dependent or may fluctuate, and some individuals with UPD remain cognitively intact despite rather severe depression. An important issue in evaluating patients with depression is their level of motivation and effort at the time of neuropsychologic testing, because adequate effort is required for obtaining valid test results.

Although studies have been somewhat inconsistent concerning reports of the nature and extent of cognitive dysfunction in BPD, a recent review of the literature indicated that deficits in executive function, verbal fluency, attention, and memory were most commonly reported [12,13]. Deficits in aspects of learning and episodic memory have been reported with some frequency in BPD, with greater deficits than in patients with UPD [2]. In addition, greater deterioration in memory functioning over time has been reported in BPD compared with UPD [14]. It has been suggested that verbal learning and memory impairments in BPD might represent cognitive trait markers of the illness, and differential scores on recall and recognition measures of verbal learning have been shown to distinguish among BPD, UPD, and non-psychiatric controls [15]. Although delayed free recall may be impaired in some cases, memory performance in BPD and UPD tends to improve when patients are provided with memory cues or when tested with a recognition format, which is a hallmark cognitive feature of subcortical system dysfunction. Despite such observations, no single cognitive profile characterizes all patients with BPD, and other differences in patterns and levels of cognitive impairment have been reported in comparisons of BPD and UPD populations [2,16–18].

Deficits in visuospatial versus verbal functioning have long been reported in association with BPD [18,19], although this finding also is not universal. In contrast, patients with schizophrenia tend to show greater deficits on verbal-oriented measures, thereby providing some additional information which may be of assistance in some challenging differential diagnostic situations [20,21]. Simple tests of visuospatial orientation do not differentiate BPD and controls as effectively as higher-order visuospatial tasks that require skills for pattern analysis and abstract reasoning [2,22]. Morice et al [23] reported that cognitive inflexibility and prefrontal cortical dysfunction may distinguish persons with BPD from normal individuals but not necessarily separate BPD from UPD, and it has been reported that subgroups of BPD patients may exist who demonstrate different levels and patterns of neurocognitive performance [18,24,25].

Such findings underscore the notion that the choice of particular neurocognitive assessment instruments may be an important factor in elucidating the presence and nature of cognitive dysfunction in BPD. In fact, the use of different cognitive assessment tools (in addition to different patient populations, clinical states, and selection criteria) may explain some of the inconsistent reports in the literature regarding the nature of cognitive dysfunction in BPD.

Cognitive function in euthymic bipolar disorder patients

Disruption of neurocognitive function during acute manic or depressed states is not surprising, although as noted, some impairments have been posited as possible trait markers. Some had assumed that remission (ie, asymptomatic periods between affective episodes) was associated with cognitive normalization in BPD. A number of studies of BPD patients during euthymic states have shed light on this issue. van Gorp et al [26] reported that euthymic BPD patients showed significant impairment on a test of verbal learning and episodic or declarative memory (the California Verbal Learning Test, a test sensitive to temporohippocampal dysfunction) but were not impaired on tests of procedural memory (which depend more upon basal ganglia integrity). Other dysfunctions reported in euthymic BPD patients include problems with attention/concentration, visuospatial organization, verbal fluency, reasoning, and problem solving [27–33]. Although not all individual patients with BPD show evidence of cognitive impairment, BPD patients as a group do tend to show lower-than-average performances on a variety of neurocognitive measures.

In summary, there are similarities and differences in cognitive dysfunction and patterns of deficits in BPD and UPD. Both groups often show deficits in learning and memory, sustained concentration, executive functions, and visuospatial abilities, although the most consistent neuropsychologic findings are problems with executive functions and episodic memory [13,34]. These deficits tend to be present regardless of mood state, suggesting that such features represent core elements of the illness and that the frontal, temporal, and subcortical systems are involved.

General factors influencing cognition in bipolar disorder

Research into cognitive functions in BPD has indicated a relationship between the degree of cognitive dysfunction and patients' age and disease severity/chronicity. For example, BPD patients who are more symptomatic, psychotic, chronically ill, and elderly tend to have greater and more diffuse cognitive impairment [22,27]. It has also been posited that, as is the case with repeated major motor seizures in epilepsy, repeated episodes of depression and (to a lesser extent) mania may have a cumulative effect on the brain, resulting in greater cognitive impairment. For example, Tham et al [35] reported that the number of hospitalizations was negatively correlated with intelligence in BPD, and van Gorp et al [26] noted that number of mood episodes (mania or depression) was negatively correlated with cognition. Kessing [36] showed that the number of depressed, but not manic or mixed episodes, was correlated most closely with cognitive deficits. It also has been observed that severity of prior course of illness in BPD, along with higher numbers of affective episodes, was associated with lower cognitive perform-ance [37]. This finding has been discussed in relation to the negative neuro-chemical cascade during affective episodes [38].

Prior course of illness and poor psychosocial functioning have been associated with reduced neurocognitive performance in a number of investi-gations [26,27,29,32,37,39,40]. Nevertheless, reduced cognitive functioning has been observed in many BPD patients during the euthymic state and in patients with childhood-onset BPD [41], thereby suggesting a core neuro-cognitive trait that may, in some cases, worsen over time, particularly with repeated affective episodes. This possibility is underscored further by studies that have found subtle cognitive inefficiencies among first-degree relatives of BPD patients [42]. Identifying which individuals may be susceptible to cognitive impairment and decline over time is an important area of future investigation, as is the identification of potential neuroprotective factors, a topic that is discussed in more detail elsewhere in this issue.

Effect of selected medications on cognition

Discussion of medication effects on cognition functions in BPD should be prefaced with the caveat that research in this area is constrained by the phenomenology of BPD. More studies specifically designed to investigate the effects of different medications on neuropsychologic functioning in BPD are needed to tease out the effects of medication on cognition. Although it is known that some medications can have negative neurocognitive side effects, a full discussion on this topic is beyond the scope of this article. Never-theless, the consistent findings of cognitive abnormalities in BPD suggest core trait-linked deficits, and the impact of medications on neuropsycho-logic functions is probably negligible [24].

Mood stabilizers

Treatment studies initially suggested that lithium had an adverse effect on attention, short-term memory, and psychomotor skills, at least among BPD patients who had been treated long term [43]. This belief seemed to be a general consensus in the field, although many patients did not report such problems subjectively [44]. More recently, however, reports have not supported the notion that lithium is necessarily detrimental to cognitive functioning in BPD [44,45].

Anticonvulsants

Historically, anticonvulsant medications have shown some success in the treatment of BPD, although the specific mechanisms of action in symptom control remain unclear. Valproate and carbamazepine were noted initially to be associated with deficits in attention, memory, and information processing, although this association remains inconclusive based upon a review of the literature [45]. A recent retrospective study of the efficacy of lamotrigine (a newer anticonvulsant) in BPD found an association with improved cognitive function [44], and the patients who showed the greatest improvement were those who were more depressed at baseline.

Atypical antipsychotics and other medications

Among patients with schizophrenia, cognitive benefits have been shown with atypical antipsychotic medications; improvements in verbal fluency, psychomotor speed and verbal memory have been associated with clozapine treatment [45,46]. Quetiapine and olanzapine have also been shown to have some beneficial cognitive and neuroprotective effect in this population [45]. Less work has been done concerning the effects of atypical antipsychotics in BPD, although risperidone has been shown to improve aspects of executive function and occupational outcomes in BPD [47].

Other classes of drugs, such as stimulants and antidepressant medications, have been tried with lesser success in improving noncognitive symptoms in BPD. Antidepressants generally are not considered to have major cognitive side effects, and some investigators have suggested that some antidepressants may have neuroprotective qualities. In a treatment study of BPD, mifepristone (RU-486), a cortisol synthesis inhibitor, was found to improve verbal fluency compared with placebo but had no significant effect on working or verbal episodic memory [48]. Furthermore, because higher cortisol levels have been found in more severe mood disorder [49], such findings may suggest a neuroprotective effect for such medications.

Methodologic issues in bipolar disorder cognition research

Some investigators have suggested that the disparate findings across studies of cognition in BPD result from the different clinical states of subjects and a lack of generalizability because of generally small sample sizes [13,22,50,51]. Additional issues include the varying methods of defining and measuring mood states and of defining remission. The lack of uniformity in the means used to evaluate cognitive functions in individuals is another factor contributing to the difficulties in studying cognition in BPD. Different tests or combinations of tests that tap different abilities have been used. Some studies use standardized neurocognitive measures that have been well validated in a variety of patient populations; others use experimental procedures that may not have normative reference data available. Last, diagnostic procedures may play a role in the variability of cognitive results across studies, because the diagnosis of BPD can be challenging, particularly early in the course of illness.

Neuroanatomic correlates of cognition in bipolar disorder

Generally, involvement of the frontal systems, (the anterior cingulate, basal ganglia, and temporolimbic systems) has been implicated in the affective disorders [9,22,52]. Enlargement of the cerebral ventricles has been reported in BPD, although this finding has also been consistent in schizophrenia [53], thereby raising the possibility that ventricular enlargement is a nonspecific feature shared with other major neuropsychiatric disorders. White-matter hyperintensities have been found to be more common in BPD than in the schizophrenias or other affective disorders [54], and general associations between these findings and neurocognitive status have also been reported. Reduced performance on measures of information-processing speed has been particularly noted in association with white-matter abnormalities in BPD [22,54].

Coffman et al [55] found impairment in a sample of psychotic bipolar patients whose deficits were correlated with a reduction in midsagittal brain areas. Sax et al [56] found that reduced prefrontal and hippocampal volumes were associated with poor performance on attentional measures in a group of manic BPD patients. It has been suggested that attention may be particularly impaired in manic BPD patients when there are abnormalities in fronto-subcortical circuits [22].

Future research direction: cognitive trait markers of bipolar disorder

Impetus for identifying cognitive trait markers for BPD stems from the finding that BPD patients, as a group, tend to demonstrate cognitive deficits, regardless of mood state. Learning and memory, sustained concentration, executive functions, and visuospatial skills are the areas in which the most consistent reductions in cognitive performance are seen, although not all BPD patients show evidence of cognitive impairment. (Also, when neuropsychiatric groups score below controls on a given task, interpretation of the level of functioning or deficit must consider whether those scores fall within or outside normal limits. In such comparisons, normative reference scores from standardized tests may be quite useful.)

Because of these factors, and because patterns of cognitive dysfunction have shown some variability across studies, interest has grown in the identification of cognitive trait vulnerability markers of BPD. Dixon et al [57], for example, suggested that specific executive-function deficits might be more intrinsic to BPD than other symptoms or particular cognitive profiles. These authors posited deficits in response initiation, strategic thinking, and inhibitory control as potential markers of BPD. Clark et al [58] proposed that deficits in sustained attention merit further investigation as a potential neurocognitive vulnerability marker for BPD [59,60]. Deficits in verbal learning and memory as reported by van Gorp et al [26] have also been suggested as potential trait markers of BPD [15,60], and others such as Glahn et al [34] have begun to explore the role of neurocognitive studies in relation to genetic analyses. A promising approach is the exploration of possible cognitive phenotypes in relatives of BPD patients to identify potential neuropsychologic markers or predictors of the later development of BPD. If reliable neurocognitive markers could be established, even within subgroups of BPD, such information might be combined with genetic, neurophysiologic, and neuroimaging results to begin to develop brain–behavior–based algorithms for the phenotypic characterization and pre-diction of treatment response in BPD and other neuropsychiatric disorders.

Summary

BPD is often associated with cognitive deficits that tend to be present regardless of mood state. Greater impairments tend to be seen in BPD patients who are older, have an early onset of the disease, and suffer a more severe course of illness. The literature also suggests that cognitive deficits are present early in patients with BPD and may be cumulative, showing an association with the number of affective (particularly depressed) episodes over time.

Cognitive deficits in BPD may share some common characteristics with those seen in patients with schizophrenia, although the latter tend to show much greater and generalized cognitive impairment. For example, unlike patients with schizophrenia, patients with BPD typically do not score lower than normal persons on measures of global intellectual ability [61]. There also is not overwhelming evidence of laterality or localization of cognitive deficits in BPD, although debate in the literature continues. More visuospatial deficits tend to be found in BPD and UPD than in schizophrenia, thereby raising the possibility of greater involvement of right hemisphere systems in mood disorders. In general, despite variability across investigations, deficits in executive functioning, episodic memory, sustained concentration, and, to a lesser extent, visuospatial skills seem to be the most consistent areas of impairment in BPD.

Just as neuroimaging anomalies have been well documented in schizophrenia, structural brain abnormalities have been noted in BPD, most commonly involving the basal ganglia or white matter [22,62–65]. Specific comparisons of cerebral atrophy and ventricular size between patients with schizophrenia and BPD have not been definitive, making it difficult to draw conclusions about structural brain abnormalities that might be specific to BPD. Nonetheless, there is enough evidence to suggest that white-matter abnormalities are reported with a greater frequency in BPD patients than in patients with UPD or schizophrenia. Functional neuro-imaging studies of mood disorders have indicated that the frontal cortex, basal ganglia, and temporal lobes are involved.

The relationships between neuroimaging and neurocognitive abnormalities in BPD are worthy of additional investigation [66]. Clearly, efforts directed toward phenotyping neuropsychiatric disorders using such measures, in addition to other clinical, neuroimaging, neurophysiologic, and genotypic information, may yield important insights into the development, nature, and course of illness. It is hoped that this understanding will lead to better identification of individuals who may be prone to greater cognitive impairment or decline and those who might be more responsive to specific treatments.

References

[1] American Psychiatric Association. Diagnostic and Statistical Manual of Mental Disorders. 4th edition. Washington (DC): American Psychiatric Association; 1994.

[2] Tavares JV, Drevets WC, Sahakian BJ. Cognition in mania and depression. Psychol Med 2003;33:959–67.

[3] Assessment. Neuropsychological testing of adults. Considerations for neurologists. Report of the Therapeutics and Technology Assessment Subcommittee of the American Academy of Neurology. Neurology 1996;47:592–9.

[4] Naugle R, Cullum CM, Bigler ED. Introduction to clinical neuropsychology: a casebook. Austin (TX): Pro-Ed; 1998.

[5] Lezak MD. Neuropsychological assessment. New York: Oxford University Press; 1994.

[6] Flashman LA, Green MF. Review of cognition and brain structure in schizophrenia: profiles, longitudinal course, and effects of treatment. Psychiatr Clin North Am 2004;27: 1–18.

[7] Docherty NM, Hawkins KA, Hoffman RE, et al. Working memory, attention, and communication disturbances in schizophrenia. J Abnorm Psychol 1996;105:212–9.

[8] Green MF, Nuechterlein KH, Gold JM, et al. Approaching a consensus cognitive battery for clinical trials in schizophrenia: the NIMH-MATRICS conference to select cognitive domains and test criteria. Biol Psychiatry 2004;56:301–7.

[9] Mayberg HS. Modulating dysfunctional limbic-cortical circuits in depression: towards development of brain-based algorithms for diagnosis and optimized treatment. Br Med Bull 2003;65:193–207.

[10] Liotti M, Mayberg HS. The role of functional neuroimaging in the neuropsychology of depression. J Clin Exp Neuropsychol 2001;23:121–36.

[11] Shenal BV, Harrison DW, Demaree HA. The neuropsychology of depression: a literature review and preliminary model. Neuropsychol Rev 2003;13:33–42.

[12] Malhi GS, Ivanovski B, Szekeres V, et al. Bipolar disorder: it's all in your mind? The neuropsychological profile of a biological disorder. Can J Psychiatry 2004;49:813–9.

[13] Deckersbach T, Savage CR, Reilly-Harrington N, et al. Episodic memory impairment in bipolar disorder and obsessive-compulsive disorder: the role of memory strategies. Bipolar Disord 2004;6:233–44.

[14] Burt T, Prudic J, Peyser S, et al. Learning and memory in bipolar and unipolar major depression: effects of aging. Neuropsychiatry Neuropsychol Behav Neurol 2000;13:246–53.

[15] Cavanagh JT, Van Beck M, Muir W, et al. Case-control study of neurocognitive function in euthymic patients with bipolar disorder: an association with mania. Br J Psychiatry 2002; 180:320–6.

[16] McGrath J, Scheldt S, Welham J, et al. Performance on tests sensitive to impaired executive ability in schizophrenia, mania and well controls: acute and subacute phases. Schizophr Res 1997;26:127–37.

[17] Sweeney JA, Kmiec JA, Kupfer DJ. Neuropsychologic impairments in bipolar and unipolar mood disorders on the CANTAB neurocognitive battery. Biol Psychiatry 2000;48:674–84.

[18] Borkowska A, Rybakowski JK. Neuropsychological frontal lobe tests indicate that bipolar depressed patients are more impaired than unipolar. Bipolar Disord 2001;3:88–94.

[19] El Badri SM, Ashton CH, Moore PB, et al. Electrophysiological and cognitive function in young euthymic patients with bipolar affective disorder. Bipolar Disord 2001;3:79–87.

[20] Goldberg TE, Gold JM, Greenberg R, et al. Contrasts between patients with affective disorders and patients with schizophrenia on a neuropsychological test battery. Am J Psychiatry 1993;150:1355–62.

[21] Hawkins KA, Hoffman RE, Quinlan DM, et al. Cognition, negative symptoms, and diagnosis: a comparison of schizophrenic, bipolar, and control samples. J Neuropsychiatry Clin Neurosci 1997;9:81–9.

[22] Bearden CE, Hoffman KM, Cannon TD. The neuropsychology and neuroanatomy of bipolar affective disorder: a critical review. Bipolar Disord 2001;3:106–50.

[23] Morice R. Cognitive inflexibility and pre-frontal dysfunction in schizophrenia and mania. Br J Psychiatry 1990;157:50–4.

[24] Altshuler LL, Ventura J, van Gorp WG, et al. Neurocognitive function in clinically stable men with bipolar I disorder or schizophrenia and normal control subjects. Biol Psychiatry 2004;56:560–9.

[25] Martinez-Aran A, Vieta E, Colom F, et al. Cognitive dysfunctions in bipolar disorder: evidence of neuropsychological disturbances. Psychother Psychosom 2000;69:2–18.

[26] van Gorp WG, Altshuler L, Theberge DC, et al. Cognitive impairment in euthymic bipolar patients with and without prior alcohol dependence. A preliminary study. Arch Gen Psychiatry 1998;55:41–6.

[27] Atre-Vaidya N, Taylor MA, Seidenberg M, et al. Cognitive deficits, psychopathology, and psychosocial functioning in bipolar mood disorder. Neuropsychiatry Neuropsychol Behav Neurol 1998;11:120–6.

[28] Hoff AL, Shukla S, Cook BL, et al. Cognitive function in manics with associated neurologic factors. J Affect Disord 1988;14:251–5.

[29] Martinez-Aran A, Vieta E, Colom F, et al. Cognitive impairment in euthymic bipolar patients: implications for clinical and functional outcome. Bipolar Disord 2004;6:224–32.

[30] Rossi A, Arduini L, Daneluzzo E, et al. Cognitive function in euthymic bipolar patients, stabilized schizophrenic patients, and healthy controls. J Psychiatr Res 2000;34:333–9.

[31] Rubinsztein JS, Michael A, Paykel ES, et al. Cognitive impairment in remission in bipolar affective disorder. Psychol Med 2000;30:1025–36.

[32] Scott J, Stanton B, Garland A. Cognitive vulnerability in patients with bipolar disorder. Psychol Med 2000;30:467–72.

[33] Ferrier IN, Stanton BR, Kelly TP, et al. Neuropsychological function in euthymic patients with bipolar disorder. Br J Psychiatry 1999;175:246–51.

[34] Glahn DC, Bearden CE, Niendam TA, et al. The feasibility of neuropsychological endophenotypes in the search for genes associated with bipolar affective disorder. Bipolar Disord 2004;6:171–82.

[35] Tham A, Engelbrektson K, Mathe AA, et al. Impaired neuropsychological performance in euthymic patients with recurring mood disorders. J Clin Psychiatry 1997;58:26–9.

[36] Kessing LV. Cognitive impairment in the euthymic phase of affective disorder. Psychol Med 1998;28:1027–38.

[37] Denicoff KD, Ali SO, Mirsky AF, et al. Relationship between prior course of illness and neuropsychological functioning in patients with bipolar disorder. J Affect Disord 1999;56: 67–73.

[38] Altshuler LL. Bipolar disorder: are repeated episodes associated with neuroanatomic and cognitive changes? Biol Psychiatry 1993;33:563–5.

[39] Dickerson FB, Boronow JJ, Stallings CR, et al. Association between cognitive functioning and employment status of persons with bipolar disorder. Psychiatr Serv 2004;55:54–8.

[40] van Gorp WG, Altshuler L, Theberge DC, et al. Declarative and procedural memory in bipolar disorder. Biol Psychiatry 1999;46:525–31.

[41] Dickstein DP, Treland JE, Snow J, et al. Neuropsychological performance in pediatric bipolar disorder. Biol Psychiatry 2004;55:32–9.

[42] Ferrier IN, Chowdhury R, Thompson JM, et al. Neurocognitive function in unaffected first-degree relatives of patients with bipolar disorder: a preliminary report. Bipolar Disord 2004; 6:319–22.

[43] Lund Y, Nissen M, Rafaelsen OJ. Long-term lithium treatment and psychological functions. Acta Psychiatr Scand 1982;65:233–44.

[44] Khan A, Ginsberg LD, Asnis GM, et al. Effect of lamotrigine on cognitive complaints in patients with bipolar I disorder. J Clin Psychiatry 2004;65:1483–90.

[45] Macqueen G, Young T. Cognitive effects of atypical antipsychotics: focus on bipolar spectrum disorders. Bipolar Disord 2003;5(Suppl 2):53–61.

[46] Sumiyoshi T, Roy A, Kim CH, et al. Prediction of changes in memory performance by plasma homovanillic acid levels in clozapine-treated patients with schizophrenia. Psychopharmacology (Berl) 2004;177:79–83.

[47] Reinares M, Martinez-Aran A, Colom F, et al. [Long-term effects of the treatment with risperidone versus conventional neuroleptics on the neuropsychological performance of euthymic bipolar patients.] Actas Esp Psiquiatr 2000;28:231–8.

[48] Young AH, Gallagher P, Watson S, et al. Improvements in neurocognitive function and mood following adjunctive treatment with mifepristone (RU-486) in bipolar disorder. Neuropsychopharmacology 2004;29:1538–45.

[49] Brown ES, Bobadilla L, Rush AJ. Ketoconazole in bipolar patients with depressive symptoms: a case series and literature review. Bipolar Disorder 2001;3(1):23–9.

[50] Murphy FC, Sahakian BJ. Neuropsychology of bipolar disorder. Br J Psychiatry 2001;178: S120–7.

[51] Quraishi S, Frangou S. Neuropsychology of bipolar disorder: a review. J Affect Disord 2002; 72:209–26.

[52] Drevets WC, Price JL, Simpson JR Jr, et al. Subgenual prefrontal cortex abnormalities in mood disorders. Nature 1997;386:824–7.

[53] Pearlson GD. Structural and functional brain changes in bipolar disorder: a selective review. Schizophr Res 1999;39:133–40.

[54] Swayze VW, Andreasen NC, Alliger RJ, et al. Structural brain abnormalities in bipolar affective disorder. Ventricular enlargement and focal signal hyperintensities. Arch Gen Psychiatry 1990;47:1054–9.

[55] Coffman JA, Bornstein RA, Olson SC, et al. Cognitive impairment and cerebral structure by MRI in bipolar disorder. Biol Psychiatry 1990;27:1188–96.

[56] Sax KW, Strakowski SM, Zimmerman ME, et al. Frontosubcortical neuroanatomy and the continuous performance test in mania. Am J Psychiatry 1999;156:139–41.

[57] Dixon T, Kravariti E, Frith C, et al. Effect of symptoms on executive function in bipolar illness. Psychol Med 2004;34:811–21.

[58] Clark L, Iversen SD, Goodwin GM. Sustained attention deficit in bipolar disorder. Br J Psychiatry 2002;180:313–9.

[59] Harmer CJ, Clark L, Grayson L, et al. Sustained attention deficit in bipolar disorder is not a working memory impairment in disguise. Neuropsychologia 2002;40:1586–90.

[60] Zalla T, Joyce C, Szoke A, et al. Executive dysfunctions as potential markers of familial vulnerability to bipolar disorder and schizophrenia. Psychiatry Res 2004;121:207–17.

[61] Kluger A, Goldberg E. IQ patterns in affective disorder, lateralized and diffuse brain damage. J Clin Exp Neuropsychol 1990;12:182–94.

[62] Dupont RM, Jernigan TL, Heindel W, et al. Magnetic resonance imaging and mood disorders. Localization of white matter and other subcortical abnormalities. Arch Gen Psychiatry 1995;52(9):747–55.

[63] Jernigan TL, Archibald SL, Berhow MT, et al. Cerebral structure on MRI, part I: localization of age-related changes. Biol Psychiatry 1991;29:55–67.

[64] Moore PB, El Badri SM, Cousins D, et al. White matter lesions and season of birth of patients with bipolar affective disorder. Am J Psychiatry 2001;158:1521–4.

[65] Strakowski SM, DelBello MP, Sax KW, et al. Brain magnetic resonance imaging of structural abnormalities in bipolar disorder. Arch Gen Psychiatry 1999;56:254–60.

[66] Stern E, Silbersweig DA. Advances in functional neuroimaging methodology for the study of brain systems underlying human neuropsychological function and dysfunction. J Clin Exp Neuropsychol 2001;23:3–18.

ELSEVIER
SAUNDERS

Psychiatr Clin N Am
28 (2005) 443–467

PSYCHIATRIC
CLINICS
OF NORTH AMERICA

Magnetic Resonance Findings in Bipolar Disorder

Paolo Brambilla, MD[a,b], David C. Glahn, PhD[c],
Matteo Balestrieri, MD[a,d], Jair C. Soares, MD[e,f,*]

[a]*Section of Psychiatry, Department of Pathology and Experimental & Clinical Medicine,
University of Udine, Udine, Italy*
[b]*Verona-Udine Brain Imaging Program, InterUniversity Center for Behavioral Neuroscience,
University of Udine, Italy*
[c]*Division of Schizophrenia and Related Disorders, Department of Psychiatry,
University of Texas Health Science Center, San Antonio, TX, USA*
[d]*InterUniversity Center for Behavioral Neuroscience, University of Udine, Italy*
[e]*Division of Mood and Anxiety Disorders, University of Texas Health Science Center,
7703 Floyd Curl Drive, San Antonio, TX, USA*
[f]*South Texas Veterans Health Care System, Audie L. Murphy Division,
San Antonio, TX, USA*

Bipolar disorder is a common, lifelong illness that typically begins in late adolescence. The illness is implicated in functional impairment and represents an important risk factor for suicide [1]. Although the pathophysiology of bipolar disorder is unknown, in the last 2 decades studies with brain imaging techniques, specifically with MRI, have reported subtle structural, chemical, and functional brain changes that provide possible hints to the neurophysiologic mechanisms of the illness. Neuroimaging research in bipolar disorder may help prevent misdiagnosis and identify the neurobiologic correlates of treatment responsiveness, ultimately leading to more effective clinical and therapeutic interventions. This article reviews structural, physiologic, and functional MRI findings in bipolar disorder and suggests future strategies for investigations in this field.

This work was supported in part by MH 01736, MH068662, MH068766, UTHSCSA GCRC (M01-RR-01346), NARSAD, the Krus Endowed Chair in Psychiatry (UTHSCSA), and the Veterans Administration (VA Merit Review).

* Corresponding author. Division of Mood and Anxiety Disorders, Department of Psychiatry, University of Texas Health Science Center, 7703 Floyd Curl Drive, San Antonio, TX 78229.

E-mail address: soares@uthscsa.edu (J.C. Soares).

doi:10.1016/j.psc.2005.01.006

Structural MRI anatomic findings

Total brain volumes

Most volumetric MRI studies report no changes in measures of total brain, gray matter, and white matter volumes of patients with bipolar disorder compared with matched healthy controls [2–8]. These findings are not universal, because abnormal reduction of cortical volume has been reported in adolescents with bipolar disorder [9], in first-episode manic patients [10], in young adult manic subjects [11], and in older patients with bipolar disorder [12]. One possible explanation for these disparate results is that patients with bipolar disorder may have a more pronounced decline in total brain matter with increasing age [3]. Currently, the available results do not indicate gross cerebral atrophy in bipolar disorder, suggesting that any structural abnormalities may be present in specific brain regions.

White matter hyperintensities

Hyperintense lesions, also known as subcortical leukoencephalopathy, have been reported in periventricular white matter and in subcortical gray matter in patients with bipolar disorder. These lesions are thought to interrupt connections between different brain regions regulating mood. Although these anomalies are not completely understood, they appear as hyperintense areas in T2-weighted MRI studies and may represent areas of increased water density, possibly caused by minor vascular damage [13]. White matter hyperintensities are found in cardiovascular diseases, such as hypertension and diabetes [14,15], and increase in frequency and intensity in healthy elderly individuals [15]. Increased rates of subcortical white matter or periventricular hyperintensities have been found in patients with bipolar disorder relative to healthy controls [16–20], particularly in older patients [3,21] or patients with poor outcome measures [17,22,23], but these findings are not universal [24–30].At present, the available findings suggest that increased rates of hyperintense lesions in bipolar disorder may be related more directly to age and severity of the illness than to the diagnosis per se.

Prefrontal cortex

The prefrontal cortex has been linked to the regulation of the expression of emotional state and thus has been of interest in volumetric studies of bipolar disorder [31]. Within the prefrontal cortex, the anterior cingulate and the dorsolateral prefrontal cortex (DLPFC) are key areas regulating cognition and emotion [32,33]. The anterior cingulate (Brodmann's areas 24, 25, and 33) has extensive connections with other brain areas involved in emotional processing [34], such as amygdala, insula, thalamus, periaqueductal gray matter, and orbitofrontal cortex [35,36]. The cingulate gyrus lies between the corpus callosum and the cingulate sulcus [37]. A tiny subregion of the anterior cingulate situated ventral to the genu of the corpus callosum, called the subgenual prefrontal cortex (SGPFC) (Brodmann's area 24), is of great interest for the pathophysiology of bipolar disorder because it participates in modulating decision making, planning, and mood regulation [38,39]. The DLPFC (Brodmann's areas 9 and 46) receives projections from higher-order association centers in the temporal and parietal lobes and plays a main role in working memory and executive brain functions [40,41].

Recently, significant decreases in volume [42,43] and gray matter density [44,45] in anterior cingulate cortex, particularly in the left side, have been reported in adult bipolar patients as compared with healthy controls. Furthermore, unmedicated patients presented decreased left anterior and posterior cingulate cortices when compared with patients treated with lithium, whereas no volumetric differences were seen between lithium-treated patients and healthy controls [43]. Decreased volumes of cingulate cortex have also been recently shown in pediatric bipolar disorder [46]. Three studies reported decreased SGPFC volumes in bipolar disorder patients with a family history of affective illness as compared with healthy control subjects [47–49], although another study did not replicate this finding [50]. Post-mortem studies demonstrated synaptic abnormalities [51] and decreased neural [52,53] and glial density [54] of the anterior cingulate in bipolar disorder, supporting the hypothesis of impaired dysfunction of cingulate neural circuits in this illness. Although the authors' structural MRI work and neuropathophysiologic studies suggest that the anterior cingulate is disturbed in bipolar disorder, not all studies have found differences in the volume of cingulate cortex between bipolar patients and controls [10,11,55].

To date, no published MRI studies have explored DLPFC morphometry in bipolar disorder. However, Lopez-Larson [11] found significantly smaller superior and middle prefrontal gray matter volumes, which encompasses part of the DLPFC, in patients with bipolar disorder compared with healthy subjects. Post-mortem studies showed reduced density and size of neurons and glial cells in the DLPFC of patients with bipolar disorder [56]. In addition, DLPFC stimulation with transcranial magnetic stimulation seemed to be effective in treating refractory depression in patients with bipolar disorder [57]. These findings suggest a possible role of DLPFC in the pathophysiology of bipolar disorder and that the size and shape of the DLPFC should be investigated.

In conclusion, prefrontal cortex dysfunction plays a major role in the pathophysiology of the bipolar illness and is correlated with reduced frontal lobe size, neuropsychologic deficits [31,55], and loss of bundle coherence in prefrontal white matter tracts [58]. Based on the available MRI literature, the anterior cingulate seems to be abnormally smaller in bipolar disorder, with the SGPFC being significantly reduced in more severely ill patients with familial bipolar disorder. Future MRI studies should attempt to further clarify the role of anatomic abnormalities in the prefrontal cortex in reflecting a genetic susceptibility to develop the disorder. Such studies should recruit larger samples of patients with familial and nonfamilial bipolar disorder, unaffected family members, and matched healthy controls. Familiarity should be investigated with direct interviews with all first-degree relatives to ascertain family psychiatric history accurately. It has recently been shown that hemispheric white matter volumes, specifically in the frontal region, are significantly reduced in bipolar type I twins as compared with control twin subjects, possibly reflecting genetic factors predisposing to alterations of prefrontal lobe in bipolar disorder [59].

Temporal lobe structures

Temporal lobes

The temporal lobes, and particularly the superior temporal gyrus (STG), are believed to be a major anatomic substrate for speech, language, and phonologic/auditory processing. In patients with bipolar illness, both decreased [60,61] and increased [5] temporal lobe volumes have been reported. Most volumetric MRI studies that measured the temporal lobe as a whole and included matched healthy comparison subjects did not find significant abnormalities in bipolar disorder [5,62–66]. When the STG is delimited, most studies found that the volume of this region does not differ between bipolar patients and comparison subjects [6,65,67,68], but other studies have disagreed [64,69].

Hippocampus

The hippocampus, together with the amygdala, orbitofrontal cortex, and anterior cingulate, is thought to be part of a circuit involved in information processing and in creation of emotional and declarative memories [70]. In particular, the hippocampus is involved in the formation of declarative memory, involving conscious recollection of facts and events, and in memory consolidation, a process converting short-term memory into long-lasting memory in the neocortex [71,72].

Although there is one report of right hemisphere hippocampal volume reduction in bipolar patients [190], most studies comparing patients with bipolar disorder and matched healthy comparison subjects did not find evidence for changes in hippocampal size [31,61,62,64,67,73–75]. Because of the sensitivity of the hippocampus to the neurotoxic effects of increased glucocorticoid levels associated with stressful episodes, it is likely that loss of hippocampus neurons is more evident in psychiatric disorders related to adverse events, such as posttraumatic stress disorder, borderline personality disorder, and major depressive disorder [71,76].

Amygdala

The amygdala receives input from the frontal and temporal lobes, and has output connections to limbic areas such as hippocampus, enthorinal-cortex, thalamus, and neocortex [77]. It is believed to be the site in which emotional memory (ie, the memory of emotionally arousing events) is formed and stored [78]. The amygdala may be involved in the production of symptoms such as fear, anxiety, and dysphoria, playing a key role in neuronal loops regulating responses to emotional stimuli [79–81].

The most consistent finding in volumetric analysis of bipolar disorder is amygdala enlargement in adult patients with bipolar disorder as compared with healthy comparison subjects [67,74,82]. Smaller than normal [64] or normal amygdala size [66] has also been reported. Findings of amygdala enlargement are consistent with findings of increased cerebral blood flow and glucose metabolism in this brain structure in bipolar patients [83]. Reports of smaller amygdala volumes in children and adolescents with bipolar disorder have also been published [9,84,85]. A direct relationship between age and left amygdala volumes was found in juvenile bipolar patients, whereas there was a reverse correlation in healthy controls [84]. Theoretically, abnormal pruning mechanisms in childhood and adolescence could lead to enlargement in adulthood in bipolar disorder. Alternatively, compensatory mechanisms operating over time might be responsible for the anatomic changes in adulthood. Several authors have proposed that enlargement of the amygdala may represent a trait marker for bipolar disorder, but longitudinal MR studies in childhood-onset patients and high-risk populations are needed to characterize amygdala development in bipolar disorder further.

Basal ganglia

The basal ganglia are composed of the caudate, putamen, and globus pallidus. They are connected to cortical and limbic regions by two parallel circuits, and disruption of different nodes in this circuit could result in dysregulation of affective state or mood regulation [86,87].

Larger striatal volumes (ie, caudate and putamen) have been found in adult [2,74,75,88] and adolescent [9,89] bipolar I patients as compared with healthy subjects and in bipolar twins compared with normal monozygotic twins in a small study [90]. In one study, duration of illness was associated with reduced volume in the lenticular nuclei (ie, putamen and globus pallidus), particularly in bipolar disorder type I [91], but most investigations have not shown any significant differences in measures of caudate, putamen, or lenticular nuclei between bipolar patients and healthy controls [4,5,10,91]. Although conflicting, the available results suggest an important role for the basal ganglia in the pathophysiology of bipolar disorder, in particular in type I patients. Future longitudinal MRI studies should examine basal ganglia over time in bipolar I versus bipolar II patients to provide more definitive answers.

Thalamus

The thalamus is a relay station between cortical and subcortical brain regions, crucial for motor and cognitive coordination. The thalamus can be divided into multiple subnuclei with different patterns of connections [92–94]. The anterior nuclei is prominently connected with the hippocampus and cingulate gyrus, the mediodorsal nucleus is the main subcortical afferent to the prefrontal cortex, and the dorsomedial nucleus is a major site for serotonergic neurotransmission [95–97].

Although two independent studies did not find differences in thalamic volumes between patients with bipolar disorder and healthy subjects [10,75,98], others have reported significant thalamic enlargement in bipolar patients [4,74]. Two studies examined thalamic size in children with bipolar disorder or schizophrenia, reporting smaller thalamic volumes in adolescents [99] and larger thalamic volumes in children [100]. Currently, there are no consistent findings concerning changes in thalamic volume in bipolar disorder. Future studies with larger samples including individuals across the lifespan may help to explain the disparate findings.

Cerebellum and vermis

In addition to involvement in motor and vestibulo-ocular regulation, the cerebellum is thought to be involved in cognitive integration and modulation of mood [101]. The cerebellum has extensive connections throughout the brain through two primary pathways: the thalamic pathway to the limbic and cortical associative areas, such as dorsolateral prefrontal cortex, medial frontal cortex, anterior cingulate, and posterior hypothalamus, and the pons/red nucleus pathway to cortical associative areas [102,103]. Recently, a cerebellar cognitive affective syndrome, characterized by deficits in executive function, spatial cognition, linguistic processing, and affect regulation, has been described [104,105].

Several CT and MRI studies report smaller cerebellum and vermis in bipolar individuals as compared with controls [106–111]. These differences seem to increase with the number of affective episodes [106,112]. Findings of reduced cerebellum volume in patients with bipolar disorder are not universal, however [112–114].

Brainstem

Connections between association and cerebellar cortices are located in the brainstem region and involve neural loops that connect the red nucleus, the inferior olive, and the dentate nucleus [115,116]. Compared with healthy controls, increased locus coeruleus neuronal density [117] and enhanced raphe echogenicity [118] have been reported in bipolar individuals, possibly suggesting functional abnormalities. The only controlled MRI report investigating brainstem volumetry in bipolar disorder showed no alterations in pons, midbrain, or medulla oblongata [112].

Ventricles

Increased size of the third [10,113] and lateral [8,18,74,75,119–122] ventricles was found in controlled CT and MRI studies in bipolar individuals, especially in those with multiple episodes. Other studies, however, did not find evidence of size abnormalities for either the third or lateral ventricles [5,12,17,20,21,63,65,73,111–113,123–126]. In a meta-analysis of this literature, a moderate composite effect size for ventricular enlargement was reported in affective disorder patients compared with normal controls [127], suggesting that any existing differences would be of small to moderate magnitude. Thus, ventricular enlargement, if present in bipolar disorder, may be less severe than in schizophrenia [127] and may primarily characterize chronic patients, representing a sign of cortical atrophy [75].

Corpus callosum

The corpus callosum is a white matter midline structure that connects the two cerebral hemispheres, allowing interhemispheric communication and playing a crucial role in cognitive processes, such as sensory-motor stimulations, attention, arousal, language, and memory [128,129]. Specifically, the genu and splenium connect association areas of the prefrontal and higher-order processing temporo-parietal cortices, whereas the callosum body and isthmus connect visual, auditory, and somatosensory areas [130]. In normal development, the corpus callosum increases in size into late adolescence, primarily by myelination of higher association areas that leads to increased speed in interhemispheric information processing and related cognitive capacity [131,132].

Few studies have examined the size of corpus callosum in patients with bipolar disorder. Studies that included the corpus callosum, however, have reported decreased area and signal intensity for total corpus callosum and its subregions (ie, genu, body, isthmus, splenium) in bipolar disorder [55,133,134]. A separate study found abnormally short callosal length [135]. Taken together, these results may suggest that there is a decrease in callosal white matter density in bipolar disorder, potentially leading to reduced speed or quantity of interhemispheric connections [136,137]. Diffusion tensor imaging, which provides more refined information on white matter organization, may help clarify the nature of corpus callosum abnormalities in bipolar disorder.

Pituitary

The pituitary gland plays a key role in the neuroendocrine regulation of a large array of body functions. The production and release of hormones by the anterior and posterior pituitary are under the influence of feedback loops involving target organs such as adrenal, thyroid, gonads, hypothalamus, and hippocampus [138,139].

One study reported decreased pituitary volumes in patients with bipolar disorder, possibly reflecting dysfunction in the hypothalamic-pituitary-adrenal

(HPA) axis [140]. This finding is in consonance with reports of HPA axis dysfunction in bipolar disorder: abnormally enhanced cortisol response to the dexamethasone/corticotrophin-releasing hormone test [141] and to waking [142] in bipolar patients has recently been demonstrated. Future MRI studies with larger patient samples are needed to replicate these findings.

Magnetic resonance spectroscopy findings

Magnetic resonance spectroscopy (MRS) is a noninvasive approach that allows in vivo investigation of brain chemistry. The most commonly used spectroscopic approach is proton MRS (^{1}H MRS), which can detect N-acetylaspartate (NAA), phosphocreatine and creatine (which are high-energy phosphate metabolites), choline-containing compounds, and myo-inositol [143,144]. Other chemicals that may be detected are lactate, lipids, and amino acid neurotransmitters, such as γ-aminobutyric acid, glutamate, and glutamine. Another technique is phosphorus (^{31}P) MRS, which is able to explore cellular metabolism and energy by measuring levels of ATP, phosphocreatine, phosphomonoesters (PME), and phosphodiesters (PDE) [145].

Proton magnetic resonance spectroscopy

N-acetylaspartate

NAA is the second most abundant amino acid after glutamate in the human brain and is the most prominent peak in the proton spectrum after water. It accounts for approximately 85% of the proton signal of the N-acetyl group; N-acetylaspartylglutamate (NAAG) accounts for the remaining 15% [146]. NAA is found only in mature neurons and is thought to be a marker of neuronal integrity, viability, and activity [147,148]. Although its specific neuronal function is unclear, there are several putative roles for NAA, including involvement in de novo synthesis of fatty acids, initiation of protein synthesis, NAAG metabolism, and aspartate storage [149].

Reductions of NAA peaks have been shown in the DLPFC of adult [150,151] and juvenile bipolar patients [152,153]. Other ^{1}H MRS studies did not find any differences in prefrontal cortex (ie, DLPFC, anterior cingulate) NAA levels in adult bipolar patients [154–158]. The discrepancy in findings among adult studies may be related to medication status, because exogenous lithium may normalize NAA levels.

Reduced NAA levels have been reported in the hippocampus, bilaterally, in adult bipolar subjects [154,159], and in the cerebellar vermis in children with a mood disorder [160]. Furthermore, increased bilateral thalamic NAA levels have been shown in euthymic male patients with bipolar I disorder compared with healthy controls [161], possibly suggesting neuronal hypertrophy, reduced glial density, or abnormal synaptic or dendritic pruning. These findings are preliminary, however, and require independent replication.

Negative findings for NAA abnormalities in bipolar disorder have been reported for the basal ganglia [154,162–165], thalamus [154], and occipital lobes [154,165].

In summary, there is evidence suggesting decreased NAA levels in juvenile and adult bipolar disorder, especially in the DLPFC, possibly resulting from dendritic/synaptic maldevelopment or neural degeneration. The ^{1}H MRS literature is quite small, however, and additional studies with larger samples need to be performed.

Choline-containing compounds

The choline peak, as visualized by ^{1}H MRS, reflects cellular membrane components and is comprised, for the major part, by choline-containing molecules, including glycerophosphocholine (GPC) plus phosphorylcholine (PC), where GPC is a breakdown product of membrane phospholipids, and PC is a precursor of membrane phospholipids, and for a small part by free choline. Therefore, free choline is not reliably separated, and possible choline abnormalities may be masked by other related compounds comprised in the peak [166].

Increased levels of choline have been reported in the anterior cingulate [167] and basal ganglia [162,163,165] of adult bipolar patients compared with healthy subjects. No changes in choline-containing molecules have been found in the prefrontal cortex (ie, DFLPC, anterior cingulate) [150,151,154–158,168], basal ganglia [164], parietal lobes [169], and hippocampus [159] of adults with bipolar disorder or in the temporal or frontal lobes in children with bipolar disorder [153,160,170]. The ^{1}H MRS research conducted thus far suggests that elevated choline levels in bipolar disorder, if present, may be specific for basal ganglia, may be independent of lithium treatment, and may suggest alterations in membrane metabolism.

Myoinositol

Myoinositol plays a crucial role in the transduction of signals in the brain, acting as a second messenger and being the key intermediate of the phosphoinositol pathway and the substrate for recycling of inositol phospholipids [166].

Higher levels of myoinositol have been detected in anterior cingulate [171,172] and medial frontal gray matter [160] of children and adolescents with bipolar disorder compared with healthy controls. No abnormalities in myoinositol levels were found in the prefrontal cortex, (ie, DLPFC and anterior cingulate) of pediatric [170] or adult bipolar patients [151,154,157,167] or in the frontal and temporal lobes of lithium- or valproate-treated euthymic adults with bipolar disorder, however [173].

The ^{1}H MRS literature for myoinositol levels in bipolar disorder is conflicting, pointing out possible elevations of myoinositol levels in the anterior cingulate in pediatric bipolar disorder that do not seem to be present in adulthood. This finding may result from abnormal signal transduction during neurodevelopment, which may be normalized by lithium administration [174]. Future ^{1}H MRS should investigate the clinical correlates of myoinositol elevation and reduction resulting from lithium treatment.

Amino acid neurotransmitters

Compared with healthy controls, elevated levels of glutamine/glutamate have been shown in the prefrontal cortex (ie, DLPFC) of bipolar adults [158] and children [170]. Recently, Dager et al [156] demonstrated elevated gray matter glutamatergic and lactate levels in the cingulate gyrus of unmedicated bipolar subjects, suggesting a shift in energy redox state from oxidative phosphorylation toward glycolysis.

Phosphorus magnetic resonance spectroscopy

In ^{31}P MRS, the PME peak represents neuronal membrane phospholipid anabolism, whereas the phosphodiesters (PDE) peak reflects catabolism. The PME/PDE ratio is high during childhood and decreases progressively after late childhood, reflecting increased neuronal membrane turnover that occurs with selective synapse elimination during this period [166].

Abnormal frontal levels of PME have been observed in bipolar disorder by Kato and colleagues [175–178], with increased concentrations during mania or depression and decreased levels in euthymia. Consistent with these findings, Deicken et al [179,180] also reported decreased PME peaks in the frontal and temporal lobes of euthymic bipolar patients. In a meta-analysis of ^{31}P MRS studies [181], euthymic bipolar patients had significantly lower PME values than healthy controls, whereas depressed bipolar patients had significantly elevated PME concentrations as compared with euthymic patients. No differences in PDE levels were found between bipolar patients and healthy individuals in these studies. Normal PME concentrations have been found in the temporal lobe [173] and basal ganglia [182] of euthymic bipolar patients, mostly in patients treated with lithium or valproate. These findings may suggest that mood stabilizers may normalize the phosphoinositol second-messenger system.

These findings suggest increased frontal and temporal membrane phospholipid anabolism during the acute phases of bipolar disorder, reflecting neuronal membrane turnover caused by clinical status or by treatment effects. The PME decreases in the euthymic state of the disease may represent trait-related alterations in signal transduction or increased synapse elimination.

Abnormally low intracellular pH in euthymic bipolar patients has been suggested [175,178,182,183], particularly in frontal lobes, basal ganglia, and areas of increased white matter hyperintensity. This finding may be a nonspecific concomitant of brain insults. Nonetheless, these preliminary results warrant replication in large independent studies.

In conclusion, there are suggestions of abnormalities in NAA, myoinositol, glutamatergic, and phospholipid metabolism in the prefrontal cortex and of abnormal choline concentrations in basal ganglia. Results are tentative, because most of these findings await independent replication. Significant variability in patient population and imaging techniques makes it difficult to compare reports. For instance, the samples involved differ in age and gender distribution as well as in clinical and medication status. Such confounding variables have not always been taken into consideration for control comparison and in statistical analyses. Also, different groups often used different imaging methods and various approaches to measure and quantify the compounds. Future MRS studies should use better-standardized research approaches to investigate longitudinal samples of unmedicated high-risk subjects, first-episode patients in various mood states, unaffected family members, and matched healthy controls, to replicate the available findings, and to determine whether the alterations are markers of vulnerability for bipolar disorder or consequences of treatment or chronicity.

Neuroprotective effects of lithium

Lithium is the reference-standard drug for acute and prophylactic treatment of bipolar disorder [184,185]. Its mechanism of action has not been elucidated, but in vitro and ex vivo studies have reported that lithium has long-term neurotrophic effects and is protective against cell death by certain insults in rodent brain and in human neuronal cells [186–188]. Specifically, lithium increases the levels of important cytoprotective proteins, such as bcl-2 [189], that are involved in the regulation of apoptotic cell death, acting on mitochondria to stabilize membrane integrity and to prevent opening of the permeability transition pore that induces apoptosis [190]. Lithium also decreases the levels of specific proapoptotic proteins, such as p53 and Bax [191], and inhibits glycogen synthase kinase 3β [187,192], an enzyme implicated in regulation of various cytoskeletal processes and disease-related neuronal death. Consistently, an MRS study reported a small but significant increase of total brain NAA (5%) after 4 weeks of lithium treatment, combining concentrations from four different voxel placements (ie, right frontal, left temporal, central occipital, and left parietal lobes) in a mixed population of bipolar and healthy subjects [193]. In lithium-treated bipolar patients, significantly increased levels of NAA have been found in the DLPFC [155], temporal lobes [194], and basal ganglia [165]. Additionally, increased total brain gray matter volumes in bipolar patients have been suggested by controlled MRI studies in patients who had been treated with lithium for 4 [195] and 27 weeks [196]. Taken together, these findings provide in vivo evidence for the neuroprotective effects of lithium in the human brain, detectable with brain imaging as an increase in neutrophil volume as a possible consequence of the trophic actions of bcl-2. Although the action of bcl-2 is the most plausible and appealing explanation for the results, the osmotic effects of lithium, leading to neuron swelling and consequent increased gray matter brain volume, could not be ruled out in these studies. A purely osmotic action would also influence the white matter volume, not only the gray matter; therefore, osmotic action seems a less likely explanation.

Recently, Sassi et al [43] found a volumetric reduction in left anterior cingulate in untreated bipolar patients compared with healthy controls but found no differences between lithium-treated patients and control subjects. Brambilla et al [144], however, did not observe any significant changes in NAA concentrations in the DLPFC of healthy individuals after 4 weeks of lithium administration. This study did not confirm the possible role of lithium in modulating cortical NAA levels in healthy volunteers. Silverstone et al [197,198] also found no significant changes in brain NAA levels after lithium administration in healthy volunteers. These findings suggest that the neuroprotective effects of lithium may be region specific and disease related. Healthy individuals, however, may not respond to pharmacologic inter- ventions in the same way that patients with psychiatric illnesses do [199]. It is possible that the neuroprotective effects of lithium can be detected in abnormal brains where NAA deficits may be present, such as those of bipolar patients, but that no such effects would be present in healthy brain tissue.

Future larger MR studies should explore the putative neuroprotective effects of lithium in first- and multiple-episode patients with bipolar disorder over longer periods. Such studies will be crucial in investigating the putative neuroprotective effects of chronic lithium treatment (resulting in increase in NAA levels or gray matter in DLPFC or other brain regions) and the relationship of these changes to treatment response in bipolar disorder.

Functional magnetic resonance findings

Advances in neuroimaging techniques, particularly noninvasive MRI methods, have significantly enhanced the understanding of the functional organization of the human brain. Functional MRI (fMRI) is one of the most widely used of these methods, in part because fMRI is noninvasive and provides adequate spatial and temporal resolution. Most fMRI experiments are based on blood oxygenation level–dependant (BOLD) methods, which measure regional cerebral hemodynamics (ie, blood flow and blood oxygenation) to make indirect inferences about neural activity [200]. During brain activation, changes in the metabolic rate of oxygen are significantly smaller than changes in the rate of cerebral blood flow, leading to an increase of local blood oxygenation and resulting in the BOLD signal. Typical fMRI experiments contrast the BOLD signal associated with a sensory or cognitive challenge and a control or resting baseline. To date, BOLD fMRI techniques have been used to study functional activation of brain regions associated with emotional and executive processing in patients with bipolar disorder.

Emotional processing tasks

Emotional processing includes the cognitive abilities associated with the perception of emotion in others and the capacity to induce and regulate emotional states within oneself. To date, three fMRI experiments have reported attempts to determine differences between patients with bipolar disorder and comparison subjects in assessing the emotional state of others. Two of these studies report that patients with bipolar disorder show increased activation of ventral/medial prefrontal cortex and subcortical areas (ie, striatum, thalamus, hippocampus) in response to viewing positive or negative emotional expressions [201,202]. A separate study, however, found decreased DLPFC and increased amygdala activation when patients were asked to rate fearful faces [203]. When rating the emotional content of spoken word, Mitchell and colleagues [204] report left rather than right lateralization of temporal lobe response, particularly for the STG, in bipolar disorder. Recently, adolescents with bipolar disorder were found to have greater signal increases in the bilateral DLPFC, inferior frontal gyrus, and right insula while viewing negatively valenced pictures and greater activation in the bilateral caudate and thalamus, left middle/superior frontal gyrus, and left anterior cingulate while viewing positively valenced pictures [205]. Discrepancies between studies may result from the different emotional states studied (eg, positive/negative versus fear), the mode of stimulus presentation, age of the participants, or variations in the imaging and analysis methods applied.

To study the neural correlates of mood induction, Malhi and colleagues [206] showed emotionally charged stimuli to patients with bipolar disorder and to matched comparison subjects. In this paradigm, patients with bipolar disorder in the depressive phase of the illness overactivated the anterior cingulate cortex, subcortical limbic cortex (ie, amygdala, hypothalamus, globus pallidus), and thalamus. Similar findings were reported for hypomanic bipolar type II patients; however, relative hyperactivation in this group was limited to the caudate [207].

Taken together, these findings are consistent with the hypothesis that the neural network associated with affective processing may be disrupted in bipolar disorder. This network, which includes the prefrontal cortex (ie, DLPFC, anterior cingulate), amygdala, and striatal nodes, is complex, and the understanding of how it functions in healthy individuals is limited. Current findings, therefore, are necessarily preliminary.

Executive function tests

During a verbal fluency task [208], bipolar patients had increased prefrontal cortical activation and decreased left ventral prefrontal cortex activation while performing a color-word Stroop task [209], in comparison to healthy controls. During an attentional task, euthymic bipolar patients showed increased activation in the limbic and ventrolateral prefrontal areas, along with visual associational cortices, whereas healthy controls exhibited relatively increased activation in the fusiform gyrus and medial prefrontal cortex [210]. Compared with healthy subjects, adolescents with bipolar disorder showed greater signal increases in the bilateral anterior cingulate, left putamen, left thalamus, left DLPFC, and right inferior frontal gyrus during the visuospatial working memory test [205] and greater activation in the left putamen and thalamus during a color-naming Stroop task [211].

During motor performance tasks, patients with bipolar disorder exhibited greater activity in the primary motor area, supplementary motor area, and striatum when compared with healthy individuals [212,213]. In particular, depressed bipolar subjects failed to suppress unwanted activity in the ipsilateral right supplementary motor area, whereas manic patients failed to suppress unwanted ipsilateral activity in left and right supplementary motor area [213].

In summary, over-reactivity of the prefrontal-limbic network has been found in subjects with bipolar disorder during tasks investigating executive functions. This over-reactivity may reflect an increased baseline excitability of emotional regions in bipolar disorder. Several different tasks were used to explore various executive functions, however, so the comparisons of these fMRI reports are hampered by this high variability.

Summary

The MR findings reviewed in this article suggest structural, chemical, and functional abnormalities in specific brain regions participating in mood and cognitive regulation, such as the DLPFC, anterior cingulate, amygdala, STG, and corpus callosum in subjects with bipolar disorder. These abnormalities would represent an altered anterior-limbic network disrupting inter- and intrahemispheric communication and underlying the expression of bipolar disorder. Available studies are limited by several confounding variables, such as small and heterogeneous patient samples, differences in clinical and medication status, and cross-sectional design. It is still unclear whether abnormalities in neurodevelopment or neurodegeneration play a major role in the pathophysiology of bipolar disorder. These processes could act together in a unitary model of the disease, with excessive neuronal pruning/apoptosis during childhood and adolescence being responsible for the onset of the disorder and subsequent neurotoxic mechanisms and impaired neuroplasticity and cellular resilience being responsible for further disease progression.

Future MR studies should investigate larger samples of first-episode drug-free patients, pediatric patients, subjects at high risk for bipolar disorder, and unaffected family members longitudinally. Such a study population is crucial to examine systematically whether brain changes are present before the appearance of symptoms (eg, maldevelopment) or whether they develop afterwards, as a result of illness course (eg, neurodegeneration). These studies will also be instrumental in minimizing potentially confounding factors commonly found in adult samples, such as the effects of long-term medication, chronicity, and hospitalizations. Juvenile bipolar patients often have a strong family history of bipolar disorder. Future studies could help elucidate the relevance of brain abnormalities as reflections of genetic susceptibility to the disorder. MR studies associated with genetic, post-mortem, and neuropsychologic studies will be valuable in separating state from trait brain abnormalities and in further characterizing the genetic determinants, the neuropathologic underpinnings, and the cognitive disturbances of bipolar disorder.

References

[1] Oquendo MA, Mann JJ. Identifying and managing suicide risk in bipolar patients. J Clin Psychiatry 2001;62(Suppl 25):31–4.

[2] Aylward EH, Roberts-Twillie JV, Barta PE, et al. Basal ganglia volumes and white matter hyperintensities in patients with bipolar disorder. Am J Psychiatry 1994;151(5):687–93.

[3] Brambilla P, Harenski K, Nicoletti M, et al. Differential effects of age on brain gray matter in bipolar patients and healthy individuals. Neuropsychobiology 2001;43(4):242–7.

[4] Dupont RM, Jernigan TL, Heindel W, et al. Magnetic resonance imaging and mood disorders. Localization of white matter and other subcortical abnormalities. Arch Gen Psychiatry 1995;52(9):747–55.

[5] Harvey I, Persaud R, Ron MA, et al. Volumetric MRI measurements in bipolars compared with schizophrenics and healthy controls. Psychol Med 1994;24(3):689–99.

[6] Schlaepfer TE, Harris GJ, Tien AY, et al. Decreased regional cortical gray matter volume in schizophrenia. Am J Psychiatry 1994;151(6):842–8.

[7] Woods BT, Yurgelun-Todd D, Mikulis D, et al. Age-related MRI abnormalities in bipolar illness: a clinical study. Biol Psychiatry 1995;38(12):846–7.

[8] Zipursky RB, Seeman MV, Bury A, et al. Deficits in gray matter volume are present in schizophrenia but not bipolar disorder. Schizophr Res 1997;26(2–3):85–92.

[9] DelBello MP, Zimmerman ME, Mills NP, et al. Magnetic resonance imaging analysis of amygdala and other subcortical brain regions in adolescents with bipolar disorder. Bipolar Disord 2004;6(1):43–52.

[10] Strakowski SM, Wilson DR, Tohen M, et al. Structural brain abnormalities in first-episode mania. Biol Psychiatry 1993;33(8–9):602–9.

[11] Lopez-Larson MP, DelBello MP, Zimmerman ME, et al. Regional prefrontal gray and white matter abnormalities in bipolar disorder. Biol Psychiatry 2002;52(2):93–100.

[12] Lim KO, Rosenbloom MJ, Faustman WO, et al. Cortical gray matter deficit in patients with bipolar disorder. Schizophr Res 1999;40(3):219–27.

[13] Fazekas F, Kleinert R, Offenbacher H, et al. The morphologic correlate of incidental punctate white matter hyperintensities on MR images. AJNR Am J Neuroradiol 1991; 12(5):915–21.

[14] Fukuda H, Kitani M. Differences between treated and untreated hypertensive subjects in the extent of periventricular hyperintensities observed on brain MRI. Stroke 1995;26(9): 1593–7.

[15] Ylikoski A, Erkinjuntti T, Raininko R, et al. White matter hyperintensities on MRI in the neurologically nondiseased elderly. Analysis of cohorts of consecutive subjects aged 55 to 85 years living at home. Stroke 1995;26(7):1171–7.

[16] Dupont RM, Jernigan TL, Butters N, et al. Subcortical abnormalities detected in bipolar affective disorder using magnetic resonance imaging. Clinical and neuropsychological significance [see comments]. Arch Gen Psychiatry 1990;47(1):55–9.

[17] Dupont RM, Jernigan TL, Gillin JC, et al. Subcortical signal hyperintensities in bipolar patients detected by MRI. Psychiatry Res 1987;21(4):357–8.

[18] Figiel GS, Krishnan KR, Rao VP, et al. Subcortical hyperintensities on brain magnetic resonance imaging: a comparison of normal and bipolar subjects. J Neuropsychiatry Clin Neurosci 1991;3(1):18–22.

[19] McDonald WM, Tupler LA, Marsteller FA, et al. Hyperintense lesions on magnetic resonance images in bipolar disorder. Biol Psychiatry 1999;45(8):965–71.

[20] Swayze VWd, Andreasen NC, Alliger RJ, et al. Structural brain abnormalities in bipolar affective disorder. Ventricular enlargement and focal signal hyperintensities. Arch Gen Psychiatry 1990;47(11):1054–9.

[21] McDonald WM, Krishnan KR, Doraiswamy PM, et al. Occurrence of subcortical hyperintensities in elderly subjects with mania. Psychiatry Res 1991;40(4):211–20.

[22] Dupont RM, Butters N, Schafer K, et al. Diagnostic specificity of focal white matter abnormalities in bipolar and unipolar mood disorder. Biol Psychiatry 1995;38(7):482–6.

[23] Moore PB, Shepherd DJ, Eccleston D, et al. Cerebral white matter lesions in bipolar affective disorder: relationship to outcome. Br J Psychiatry 2001;178:172–6.

[24] Botteron KN, Vannier MW, Geller B, et al. Preliminary study of magnetic resonance imaging characteristics in 8- to 16-year-olds with mania. J Am Acad Child Adolesc Psychiatry 1995;34(6):742–9.

[25] Brown FW, Lewine RJ, Hudgins PA, et al. White matter hyperintensity signals in psychiatric and nonpsychiatric subjects. Am J Psychiatry 1992;149(5):620–5.

[26] Krabbendam L, Honig A, Wiersma J, et al. Cognitive dysfunctions and white matter lesions in patients with bipolar disorder in remission. Acta Psychiatr Scand 2000;101(4):274–80.

[27] Persaud R, Russow H, Harvey I, et al. Focal signal hyperintensities in schizophrenia. Schizophr Res 1997;27(1):55–64.

[28] Sassi RB, Brambilla P, Nicoletti M, et al. White matter hyperintensities in bipolar and unipolar patients with relatively mild-to-moderate illness severity. J Affect Disord 2003; 77(3):237–45.

[29] Silverstone T, McPherson H, Li Q, et al. Deep white matter hyperintensities in patients with bipolar depression, unipolar depression and age-matched control subjects. Bipolar Disord 2003;5(1):53–7.

[30] Strakowski SM, Woods BT, Tohen M, et al. MRI subcortical signal hyperintensities in mania at first hospitalization. Biol Psychiatry 1993;33(3):204–6.

[31] Sax KW, Strakowski SM, Zimmerman ME, et al. Frontosubcortical neuroanatomy and the continuous performance test in mania. Am J Psychiatry 1999;156(1):139–41.

[32] Gray JR, Braver TS, Raichle ME. Integration of emotion and cognition in the lateral prefrontal cortex. Proc Natl Acad Sci U S A 2002;99(6):4115–20.

[33] Teasdale JD, Howard RJ, Cox SG, et al. Functional MRI study of the cognitive generation of affect. Am J Psychiatry 1999;156(2):209–15.

[34] Bush G, Vogt BA, Holmes J, et al. Dorsal anterior cingulate cortex: a role in reward-based decision making. Proc Natl Acad Sci U S A 2002;99(1):523–8.

[35] Barbas H. Connections underlying the synthesis of cognition, memory, and emotion in primate prefrontal cortices. Brain Res Bull 2000;52(5):319–30.

[36] Lane RD, Reiman EM, Axelrod B, et al. Neural correlates of levels of emotional awareness. Evidence of an interaction between emotion and attention in the anterior cingulate cortex. J Cogn Neurosci 1998;10(4):525–35.

[37] Vogt BA, Berger GR, Derbyshire SW. Structural and functional dichotomy of human midcingulate cortex. Eur J Neurosci 2003;18(11):3134–44.

[38] Drevets WC, Ongur D, Price JL. Neuroimaging abnormalities in the subgenual prefrontal cortex: implications for the pathophysiology of familial mood disorders. Mol Psychiatry 1998;3(3):220–6, 190–1(Review).

[39] Vogt BA, Nimchinsky EA, Vogt LJ, et al. Human cingulate cortex: surface features, flat maps, and cytoarchitecture. J Comp Neurol 1995;359(3):490–506.

[40] Cabeza R, Nyberg L. Imaging cognition II: an empirical review of 275 PET and fMRI studies. J Cogn Neurosci 2000;12(1):1–47.

[41] Smith EE, Jonides J. Storage and executive processes in the frontal lobes. Science 1999; 283(5408):1657–61.

[42] Lochhead RA, Parsey RV, Oquendo MA, et al. Regional brain gray matter volume differences in patients with bipolar disorder as assessed by optimized voxel-based morphometry. Biol Psychiatry 2004;55(12):1154–62.

[43] Sassi RB, Brambilla P, Hatch JP, et al. Reduced left anterior cingulate volumes in untreated bipolar patients. Biol Psychiatry 2004;56(7):467–75.

[44] Doris A, Belton E, Ebmeier KP, et al. Reduction of cingulate gray matter density in poor outcome bipolar illness. Psychiatry Res 2004;130(2):153–9.

[45] Lyoo IK, Kim MJ, Stoll AL, et al. Frontal lobe gray matter density decreases in bipolar I disorder. Biol Psychiatry 2004;55(6):648–51.

[46] Kaur S, Sassi RB, Axelson D, et al. Anatomical abnormalities in cingulate cortex in children and adolescents with bipolar disorder. Am J Psychiatry In press.

[47] Drevets WC, Price JL, Simpson JR Jr, et al. Subgenual prefrontal cortex abnormalities in mood disorders [see comments]. Nature 1997;386(6627):824–7.

[48] Hirayasu Y, Shenton ME, Salisbury DF, et al. Subgenual cingulate cortex volume in first-episode psychosis [in process citation]. Am J Psychiatry 1999;156(7):1091–3.

[49] Sharma V, Menon R, Carr TJ, et al. An MRI study of subgenual prefrontal cortex in patients with familial and non-familial bipolar I disorder. J Affect Disord 2003;77(2): 167–71.

[50] Brambilla P, Nicoletti MA, Harenski K, et al. Anatomical MRI study of subgenual prefrontal cortex in bipolar and unipolar subjects. Neuropsychopharmacology 2002;27(5): 792–9.

[51] Eastwood SL, Harrison PJ. Synaptic pathology in the anterior cingulate cortex in schizophrenia and mood disorders. A review and a Western blot study of synaptophysin, GAP-43 and the complexins. Brain Res Bull 2001;55(5):569–78.

[52] Benes FM, Vincent SL, Todtenkopf M. The density of pyramidal and nonpyramidal neurons in anterior cingulate cortex of schizophrenic and bipolar subjects. Biol Psychiatry 2001;50(6):395–406.

[53] Bouras C, Kovari E, Hof PR, et al. Anterior cingulate cortex pathology in schizophrenia and bipolar disorder. Acta Neuropathol (Berl) 2001;102(4):373–9.

[54] Ongur D, Drevets WC, Price JL. Glial reduction in the subgenual prefrontal cortex in mood disorders. Proc Natl Acad Sci U S A 1998;95(22):13290–5.

[55] Coffman JA, Bornstein RA, Olson SC, et al. Cognitive impairment and cerebral structure by MRI in bipolar disorder. Biol Psychiatry 1990;27(11):1188–96.

[56] Rajkowska G, Halaris A, Selemon LD. Reductions in neuronal and glial density characterize the dorsolateral prefrontal cortex in bipolar disorder. Biol Psychiatry 2001; 49(9):741–52.

[57] George L, Neufeld RW. Attentional resources and hemispheric functional asymmetry in schizophrenia. Br J Clin Psychol 1987;26(Pt 1):35–45.

[58] Adler CM, Holland SK, Schmithorst V, et al. Abnormal frontal white matter tracts in bipolar disorder: a diffusion tensor imaging study. Bipolar Disord 2004;6(3):197–203.

[59] Kieseppa T, van Erp TG, Haukka J, et al. Reduced left hemispheric white matter volume in twins with bipolar I disorder. Biol Psychiatry 2003;54(9):896–905.

[60] Altshuler LL, Conrad A, Hauser P, et al. Reduction of temporal lobe volume in bipolar disorder: a preliminary report of magnetic resonance imaging [letter]. Arch Gen Psychiatry 1991;48(5):482–3.

[61] Hauser P, Altshuler LL, Berrettini W, et al. Temporal lobe measurement in primary affective disorder by magnetic resonance imaging. J Neuropsychiatry Clin Neurosci 1989; 1(2):128–34.

[62] Altshuler LL, Bartzokis G, Grieder T, et al. Amygdala enlargement in bipolar disorder and hippocampal reduction in schizophrenia: an MRI study demonstrating neuroanatomic specificity [letter]. Arch Gen Psychiatry 1998;55(7):663–4.

[63] Johnstone EC, Owens DG, Crow TJ, et al. Temporal lobe structure as determined by nuclear magnetic resonance in schizophrenia and bipolar affective disorder. J Neurol Neurosurg Psychiatry 1989;52(6):736–41.

[64] Pearlson GD, Barta PE, Powers RE, et al. Ziskind-Somerfeld Research Award 1996. Medial and superior temporal gyral volumes and cerebral asymmetry in schizophrenia versus bipolar disorder. Biol Psychiatry 1997;41(1):1–14.

[65] Roy PD, Zipursky RB, Saint-Cyr JA, et al. Temporal horn enlargement is present in schizophrenia and bipolar disorder. Biol Psychiatry 1998;44(6):418–22.

[66] Swayze VW 2nd, Andreasen NC, Alliger RJ, et al. Subcortical and temporal structures in affective disorder and schizophrenia: a magnetic resonance imaging study [see comments]. Biol Psychiatry 1992;31(3):221–40.

[67] Brambilla P, Harenski K, Nicoletti M, et al. MRI investigation of temporal lobe structures in bipolar patients. J Psychiatr Res 2003;37(4):287–95.

[68] Hirayasu Y, Shenton ME, Salisbury DF, et al. Lower left temporal lobe MRI volumes in patients with first-episode schizophrenia compared with psychotic patients with first-episode affective disorder and normal subjects. Am J Psychiatry 1998;155(10):1384–91.

[69] Chen HH, Nicoletti MA, Hatch JP, et al. Abnormal left superior temporal gyrus volumes in children and adolescents with bipolar disorder: a magnetic resonance imaging study. Neurosci Lett 2004;363(1):65–8.

[70] Poldrack RA, Gabrieli JD. Functional anatomy of long-term memory. J Clin Neurophysiol 1997;14(4):294–310.

[71] Sala M, Perez J, Soloff P, et al. Stress and hippocampal abnormalities in psychiatric disorders. Eur Neuropsychopharmacol 2004;14(5):393–405.

[72] Wittenberg GM, Tsien JZ. An emerging molecular and cellular framework for memory processing by the hippocampus. Trends Neurosci 2002;25(10):501–5.

[73] Hauser P, Matochik J, Altshuler LL, et al. MRI-based measurements of temporal lobe and ventricular structures in patients with bipolar I and bipolar II disorders. J Affect Disord 2000;60(1):25–32.

[74] Strakowski SM, DelBello MP, Sax KW, et al. Brain magnetic resonance imaging of structural abnormalities in bipolar disorder. Arch Gen Psychiatry 1999;56(3):254–60.

[75] Strakowski SM, DelBello MP, Zimmerman ME, et al. Ventricular and periventricular structural volumes in first- versus multiple-episode bipolar disorder. Am J Psychiatry 2002; 159(11):1841–7.

[76] Brambilla P, Soloff PH, Sala M, et al. Anatomical MRI study of borderline personality disorder patients. Psychiatry Res 2004;131(2):125–33.

[77] McGaugh JL, Cahill L, Roozendaal B. Involvement of the amygdala in memory storage: interaction with other brain systems. Proc Natl Acad Sci U S A 1996;93(24):13508–14.

[78] Cahill L, Babinsky R, Markowitsch HJ, et al. The amygdala and emotional memory. Nature 1995;377(6547):295–6.

[79] Adolphs R, Baron-Cohen S, Tranel D. Impaired recognition of social emotions following amygdala damage. J Cogn Neurosci 2002;14(8):1264–74.

[80] Morris JS, Frith CD, Perrett DI, et al. A differential neural response in the human amygdala to fearful and happy facial expressions. Nature 1996;383(6603):812–5.

[81] Schneider F, Grodd W, Weiss U, et al. Functional MRI reveals left amygdala activation during emotion. Psychiatry Res 1997;76(2–3):75–82.

[82] Altshuler LL, Bartzokis G, Grieder T, et al. An MRI study of temporal lobe structures in men with bipolar disorder or schizophrenia. Biol Psychiatry 2000;48(2):147–62.

[83] Drevets WC. Prefrontal cortical-amygdalar metabolism in major depression [in process citation]. Ann N Y Acad Sci 1999;877:614–37.

[84] Chen BK, Sassi R, Axelson D, et al. Cross-sectional study of abnormal amygdala development in adolescents and young adults with bipolar disorder. Biol Psychiatry 2004; 56(6):399–405.

[85] Blumberg HP, Kaufman J, Martin A, et al. Amygdala and hippocampal volumes in adolescents and adults with bipolar disorder. Arch Gen Psychiatry 2003;60(12):1201–8.

[86] Alexander GE, DeLong MR, Strick PL. Parallel organization of functionally segregated circuits linking basal ganglia and cortex. Annu Rev Neurosci 1986;9:357–81.

[87] Mega MS, Cummings JL. Frontal-subcortical circuits and neuropsychiatric disorders. J Neuropsychiatry Clin Neurosci 1994;6(4):358–70.

[88] Getz GE, DelBello MP, Fleck DE, et al. Neuroanatomic characterization of schizoaffective disorder using MRI: a pilot study. Schizophr Res 2002;55(1–2):55–9.

[89] Wilke M, Kowatch RA, DelBello MP, et al. Voxel-based morphometry in adolescents with bipolar disorder: first results. Psychiatry Res 2004;131(1):57–69.

[90] Noga JT, Vladar K, Torrey EF. A volumetric magnetic resonance imaging study of monozygotic twins discordant for bipolar disorder. Psychiatry Res 2001;106(1):25–34.

[91] Brambilla P, Harenski K, Nicoletti MA, et al. Anatomical MRI study of basal ganglia in bipolar disorder patients. Psychiatry Res 2001;106(2):65–80.

[92] Macchi G, Jones EG. Toward an agreement on terminology of nuclear and subnuclear divisions of the motor thalamus. J Neurosurg 1997;86(4):670–85.

[93] Price JL. Prefrontal cortical networks related to visceral function and mood. Ann N Y Acad Sci 1999;877:383–96.

[94] Rodriguez A, Whitson J, Granger R. Derivation and analysis of basic computational operations of thalamocortical circuits. J Cogn Neurosci 2004;16(5):856–77.

[95] Guye M, Parker GJ, Symms M, et al. Combined functional MRI and tractography to demonstrate the connectivity of the human primary motor cortex in vivo. Neuroimage 2003;19(4):1349–60.

[96] Spinks R, Magnotta VA, Andreasen NC, et al. Manual and automated measurement of the whole thalamus and mediodorsal nucleus using magnetic resonance imaging. Neuroimage 2002;17(2):631–42.

[97] Van der Werf YD, Witter MP, Groenewegen HJ. The intralaminar and midline nuclei of the thalamus. Anatomical and functional evidence for participation in processes of arousal and awareness. Brain Res Brain Res Rev 2002;39(2–3):107–40.

[98] Caetano SC, Sassi R, Brambilla P, et al. MRI study of thalamic volumes in bipolar and unipolar patients and healthy individuals. Psychiatry Res 2001;108(3):161–8.

[99] Dasari M, Friedman L, Jesberger J, et al. A magnetic resonance imaging study of thalamic area in adolescent patients with either schizophrenia or bipolar disorder as compared to healthy controls. Psychiatry Res 1999;91(3):155–62.

[100] Frazier JA, Giedd JN, Hamburger SD, et al. Brain anatomic magnetic resonance imaging in childhood-onset schizophrenia. Arch Gen Psychiatry 1996;53(7):617–24.

[101] Makris N, Hodge SM, Haselgrove C, et al. Human cerebellum: surface-assisted cortical parcellation and volumetry with magnetic resonance imaging. J Cogn Neurosci 2003;15(4): 584–99.

[102] Leiner HC, Leiner AL, Dow RS. Cognitive and language functions of the human cerebellum. Trends Neurosci 1993;16(11):444–7.

[103] Snider RS, Maiti A, Snider SR. Cerebellar connections to catecholamine systems: anatomical and biochemical studies. Trans Am Neurol Assoc 1976;101:295–7.

[104] Levisohn L, Cronin-Golomb A, Schmahmann JD. Neuropsychological consequences of cerebellar tumour resection in children: cerebellar cognitive affective syndrome in a paediatric population. Brain 2000;123(Pt 5):1041–50.

[105] Schmahmann JD. Disorders of the cerebellum: ataxia, dysmetria of thought, and the cerebellar cognitive affective syndrome. J Neuropsychiatry Clin Neurosci 2004;16(3): 367–78.

[106] DelBello MP, Strakowski SM, Zimmerman ME, et al. MRI analysis of the cerebellum in bipolar disorder: a pilot study [in process citation]. Neuropsychopharmacology 1999;21(1): 63–8.

[107] Lippmann S, Manshadi M, Baldwin H, et al. Cerebellar vermis dimensions on computerized tomographic scans of schizophrenic and bipolar patients. Am J Psychiatry 1982;139(5):667–8.

[108] Nasrallah HA, Jacoby CG, McCalley-Whitters M. Cerebellar atrophy in schizophrenia and mania [letter]. Lancet 1981;1(8229):1102.

[109] Nasrallah HA, McCalley-Whitters M, Jacoby CG. Cerebral ventricular enlargement in young manic males. A controlled CT study. J Affect Disord 1982;4(1):15–9.

[110] Rieder RO, Mann LS, Weinberger DR, et al. Computed tomographic scans in patients with schizophrenia, schizoaffective, and bipolar affective disorder. Arch Gen Psychiatry 1983; 40(7):735–9.

[111] Weinberger DR, DeLisi LE, Perman GP, et al. Computed tomography in schizophreniform disorder and other acute psychiatric disorders. Arch Gen Psychiatry 1982;(39):778–83.

[112] Brambilla P, Harenski K, Nicoletti M, et al. MRI study of posterior fossa structures and brain ventricles in bipolar patients. J Psychiatr Res 2001;35(6):313–22.

[113] Dewan MJ, Haldipur CV, Lane EE, et al. Bipolar affective disorder. I. Comprehensive quantitative computed tomography. Acta Psychiatr Scand 1988;77(6):670–6.

[114] Yates WR, Jacoby CG, Andreasen NC. Cerebellar atrophy in schizophrenia and affective disorder. Am J Psychiatry 1987;144(4):465–7.

[115] Inglis WL, Winn P. The pedunculopontine tegmental nucleus: where the striatum meets the reticular formation. Prog Neurobiol 1995;47(1):1–29.

[116] Schmahmann JD, Pandya DN. The cerebrocerebellar system. Int Rev Neurobiol 1997;41: 31–60.

[117] Baumann B, Danos P, Krell D, et al. Unipolar-bipolar dichotomy of mood disorders is supported by noradrenergic brainstem system morphology [in process citation]. J Affect Disord 1999;54(1–2):217–24.

[118] Becker G, Becker T, Struck M, et al. Reduced echogenicity of brainstem raphe specific to unipolar depression: a transcranial color-coded real-time sonography study. Biol Psychiatry 1995;38(3):180–4.

[119] Andreasen NC, Swayze VD, Flaum M, et al. Ventricular abnormalities in affective disorder: clinical and demographic correlates. Am J Psychiatry 1990;147(7):893–900.

[120] Lippmann S, Manshadi M, Baldwin H, et al. Cerebral CAT scan imaging in schizophrenic and bipolar patients. J Ky Med Assoc 1985;83(1):13–5.

[121] Nasrallah HA, McCalley-Whitters M, Jacoby CG. Cortical atrophy in schizophrenia and mania: a comparative CT study. J Clin Psychiatry 1982;43(11):439–41.

[122] Pearlson GD, Garbacz DJ, Breakey WR, et al. Lateral ventricular enlargement associated with persistent unemployment and negative symptoms in both schizophrenia and bipolar disorder. Psychiatry Res 1984;12(1):1–9.

[123] Iacono WG, Smith GN, Moreau M, et al. Ventricular and sulcal size at the onset of psychosis. Am J Psychiatry 1988;145(7):820–4.

[124] Risch SC, Lewine RJ, Kalin NH, et al. Limbic-hypothalamic-pituitary-adrenal axis activity and ventricular-to-brain ratio studies in affective illness and schizophrenia. Neuropsychopharmacology 1992;6(2):95–100.

[125] Schlegel S, Kretzschmar K. Computed tomography in affective disorders. Part II. Brain density. Biol Psychiatry 1987;22(1):15–23.

[126] Tanaka Y, Hazama H, Fukuhara T, et al. Computerized tomography of the brain in manic-depressive patients–a controlled study. Folia Psychiatr Neurol Jpn 1982;36(2):137–43.

[127] Elkis H, Friedman L, Wise A, et al. Meta-analyses of studies of ventricular enlargement and cortical sulcal prominence in mood disorders. Comparisons with controls or patients with schizophrenia. Arch Gen Psychiatry 1995;52(9):735–46.

[128] Hellige JB, Taylor KB, Lesmes L, et al. Relationships between brain morphology and behavioral measures of hemispheric asymmetry and interhemispheric interaction. Brain Cogn 1998;36(2):158–92.

[129] Phelps EA, Hirst W, Gazzaniga MS. Deficits in recall following partial and complete commissurotomy. Cereb Cortex 1991;1(6):492–8.

[130] Aboitiz F, Scheibel AB, Fisher RS, et al. Fiber composition of the human corpus callosum. Brain Res 1992;598(1–2):143–53.

[131] Giedd JN, Blumenthal J, Jeffries NO, et al. Development of the human corpus callosum during childhood and adolescence: a longitudinal MRI study. Prog Neuropsychopharmacol Biol Psychiatry 1999;23(4):571–88.

[132] Keshavan MS, Diwadkar VA, DeBellis M, et al. Development of the corpus callosum in childhood, adolescence and early adulthood. Life Sci 2002;70(16):1909–22.

[133] Brambilla P, Nicoletti M, Sassi RB, et al. Corpus callosum signal intensity in patients with bipolar and unipolar disorder. J Neurol Neurosurg Psychiatry 2004;75(2):221–5.

[134] Brambilla P, Nicoletti MA, Sassi RB, et al. Magnetic resonance imaging study of corpus callosum abnormalities in patients with bipolar disorder. Biol Psychiatry 2003;54(11):1294–7.

[135] Hauser P, Dauphinais ID, Berrettini W, et al. Corpus callosum dimensions measured by magnetic resonance imaging in bipolar affective disorder and schizophrenia. Biol Psychiatry 1989;26(7):659–68.

[136] El-Badri SM, Ashton CH, Moore PB, et al. Electrophysiological and cognitive function in young euthymic patients with bipolar affective disorder. Bipolar Disord 2001;3(2):79–87.

[137] Wilder-Willis KE, Sax KW, Rosenberg HL, et al. Persistent attentional dysfunction in remitted bipolar disorder. Bipolar Disord 2001;3(2):58–62.

[138] Wilson ME, Handa RJ. Activin subunit, follistatin, and activin receptor gene expression in the prepubertal female rat pituitary. Biol Reprod 1998;59(2):278–83.

[139] Wilson ME, Handa RJ. Direct actions of gonadal steroid hormones on FSH secretion and expression in the infantile female rat. J Steroid Biochem Mol Biol 1998;66(1–2):71–8.

[140] Sassi RB, Nicoletti M, Brambilla P, et al. Decreased pituitary volume in patients with bipolar disorder. Biol Psychiatry 2001;50(4):271–80.

[141] Watson S, Gallagher P, Ritchie JC, et al. Hypothalamic-pituitary-adrenal axis function in patients with bipolar disorder. Br J Psychiatry 2004;184:496–502.

[142] Deshauer D, Duffy A, Alda M, et al. The cortisol awakening response in bipolar illness: a pilot study. Can J Psychiatry 2003;48(7):462–6.

[143] Brambilla P, Stanley JA, Nicoletti M, et al. 1H MRS brain measures and acute lorazepam administration in healthy human subjects. Neuropsychopharmacology 2002;26(4):546–51.

[144] Brambilla P, Stanley JA, Sassi RB, et al. 1H MRS study of dorsolateral prefrontal cortex in healthy individuals before and after lithium administration. Neuropsychopharmacology 2004;29(10):1918–24.

[145] Soares JC, Krishnan KR, Keshavan MS. Nuclear magnetic resonance spectroscopy: new insights into the pathophysiology of mood disorders. Depression 1996;4(1):14–30.

[146] Pouwels PJ, Frahm J. Regional metabolite concentrations in human brain as determined by quantitative localized proton MRS. Magn Reson Med 1998;39(1):53–60.

[147] Simmons ML, Frondoza CG, Coyle JT. Immunocytochemical localization of N-acetyl-aspartate with monoclonal antibodies. Neuroscience 1991;45(1):37–45.

[148] Urenjak J, Williams SR, Gadian DG, et al. Proton nuclear magnetic resonance spectroscopy unambiguously identifies different neural cell types. J Neurosci 1993;13(3): 981–9.

[149] Tsai G, Coyle JT. N-acetylaspartate in neuropsychiatric disorders. Prog Neurobiol 1995; 46(5):531–40.

[150] Cecil KM, DelBello MP, Morey R, et al. Frontal lobe differences in bipolar disorder as determined by proton MR spectroscopy. Bipolar Disord 2002;4(6):357–65.

[151] Winsberg ME, Sachs N, Tate DL, et al. Decreased dorsolateral prefrontal N-acetyl aspartate in bipolar disorder. Biol Psychiatry 2000;47(6):475–81.

[152] Chang K, Adleman N, Dienes K, et al. Decreased N-acetylaspartate in children with familial bipolar disorder. Biol Psychiatry 2003;53(11):1059–65.

[153] Sassi RB, Stanley JA, Axelson D, et al. Reduced N-acetyl-aspartate levels in the dorsolateral prefrontal cortex of adolescent bipolar patients. Am J Psychiatry In press.

[154] Bertolino A, Frye M, Callicott JH, et al. Neuronal pathology in the hippocampal area of patients with bipolar disorder: a study with proton magnetic resonance spectroscopic imaging. Biol Psychiatry 2003;53(10):906–13.

[155] Brambilla P, Stanley JA, Nicoletti M, et al. 1H Magnetic resonance spectroscopy investigation of the dorsolateral prefrontal cortex in bipolar disorder patients. J Affect Disord, in press.

[156] Dager SR, Friedman SD, Parow A, et al. Brain metabolic alterations in medication-free patients with bipolar disorder. Arch Gen Psychiatry 2004;61(5):450–8.

[157] Hamakawa H, Kato T, Shioiri T, et al. Quantitative proton magnetic resonance spectroscopy of the bilateral frontal lobes in patients with bipolar disorder [in process citation]. Psychol Med 1999;29(3):639–44.

[158] Michael N, Erfurth A, Ohrmann P, et al. Acute mania is accompanied by elevated glutamate/glutamine levels within the left dorsolateral prefrontal cortex. Psychopharmacology (Berl) 2003;168(3):344–6.

[159] Deicken RF, Pegues MP, Anzalone S, et al. Lower concentration of hippocampal N-acetylaspartate in familial bipolar I disorder. Am J Psychiatry 2003;160(5): 873–82.

[160] Cecil KM, DelBello MP, Sellars MC, et al. Proton magnetic resonance spectroscopy of the frontal lobe and cerebellar vermis in children with a mood disorder and a familial risk for bipolar disorders. J Child Adolesc Psychopharmacol 2003;13(4):545–55.

[161] Deicken RF, Eliaz Y, Feiwell R, et al. Increased thalamic N-acetylaspartate in male patients with familial bipolar I disorder. Psychiatry Res 2001;106(1):35–45.

[162] Hamakawa H, Kato T, Murashita J, et al. Quantitative proton magnetic resonance spectroscopy of the basal ganglia in patients with affective disorders. Eur Arch Psychiatry Clin Neurosci 1998;248(1):53–8.

[163] Kato T, Hamakawa H, Shioiri T, et al. Choline-containing compounds detected by proton magnetic resonance spectroscopy in the basal ganglia in bipolar disorder. J Psychiatry Neurosci 1996;21(4):248–54.

[164] Ohara K, Isoda H, Suzuki Y, et al. Proton magnetic resonance spectroscopy of the lenticular nuclei in bipolar I affective disorder. Psychiatry Res 1998;84(2–3):55–60.

[165] Sharma R, Venkatasubramanian PN, Barany M, et al. Proton magnetic resonance spectroscopy of the brain in schizophrenic and affective patients. Schizophr Res 1992;8(1): 43–9.

[166] Stanley JA. In vivo magnetic resonance spectroscopy and its application to neuropsychiatric disorders. Can J Psychiatry 2002;47(4):315–26.

[167] Moore CM, Breeze JL, Gruber SA, et al. Choline, myo-inositol and mood in bipolar disorder: a proton magnetic resonance spectroscopic imaging study of the anterior cingulate cortex. Bipolar Disord 2000;2(3 Pt 2):207–16.

[168] Wu RH, O'Donnell T, Ulrich M, et al. Brain choline concentrations may not be altered in euthymic bipolar disorder patients chronically treated with either lithium or sodium valproate. Ann Gen Hosp Psychiatry 2004;3(1):13.

[169] Stoll AL, Renshaw PF, Sachs GS, et al. The human brain resonance of choline-containing compounds is similar in patients receiving lithium treatment and controls: an in vivo proton magnetic resonance spectroscopy study. Biol Psychiatry 1992;32(10):944–9.

[170] Castillo M, Kwock L, Courvoisie H, et al. Proton MR spectroscopy in children with bipolar affective disorder: preliminary observations. AJNR Am J Neuroradiol 2000;21(5):832–8.

[171] Davanzo P, Thomas MA, Yue K, et al. Decreased anterior cingulate myo-inositol/creatine spectroscopy resonance with lithium treatment in children with bipolar disorder. Neuropsychopharmacology 2001;24(4):359–69.

[172] Davanzo P, Yue K, Thomas MA, et al. Proton magnetic resonance spectroscopy of bipolar disorder versus intermittent explosive disorder in children and adolescents. Am J Psychiatry 2003;160(8):1442–52.

[173] Silverstone PH, Wu RH, O'Donnell T, et al. Chronic treatment with both lithium and sodium valproate may normalize phosphoinositol cycle activity in bipolar patients. Hum Psychopharmacol 2002;17(7):321–7.

[174] Moore GJ, Bebchuk JM, Parrish JK, et al. Temporal dissociation between lithium-induced changes in frontal lobe myo-inositol and clinical response in manic-depressive illness. Am J Psychiatry 1999;156(12):1902–8.

[175] Kato T, Shioiri T, Murashita J, et al. Phosphorus-31 magnetic resonance spectroscopy and ventricular enlargement in bipolar disorder. Psychiatry Res 1994;55(1):41–50.

[176] Kato T, Shioiri T, Takahashi S, et al. Measurement of brain phosphoinositide metabolism in bipolar patients using in vivo 31P-MRS. J Affect Disord 1991;22(4):185–90.

[177] Kato T, Takahashi S, Shioiri T, et al. Brain phosphorous metabolism in depressive disorders detected by phosphorus-31 magnetic resonance spectroscopy. J Affect Disord 1992;26(4):223–30.

[178] Kato T, Takahashi S, Shioiri T, et al. Alterations in brain phosphorous metabolism in bipolar disorder detected by in vivo 31P and 7Li magnetic resonance spectroscopy. J Affect Disord 1993;27(1):53–9.

[179] Deicken RF, Fein G, Weiner MW. Abnormal frontal lobe phosphorous metabolism in bipolar disorder. Am J Psychiatry 1995;152(6):915–8.

[180] Deicken RF, Weiner MW, Fein G. Decreased temporal lobe phosphomonoesters in bipolar disorder. J Affect Disord 1995;33(3):195–9.

[181] Yildiz A, Sachs GS, Dorer DJ, et al. 31P Nuclear magnetic resonance spectroscopy findings in bipolar illness: a meta-analysis. Psychiatry Res 2001;106(3):181–91.

[182] Hamakawa H, Murashita J, Yamada N, et al. Reduced intracellular pH in the basal ganglia and whole brain measured by 31P-MRS in bipolar disorder. Psychiatry Clin Neurosci 2004; 58(1):82–8.

[183] Kato T, Murashita J, Kamiya A, et al. Decreased brain intracellular pH measured by 31P-MRS in bipolar disorder: a confirmation in drug-free patients and correlation with white matter hyperintensity. Eur Arch Psychiatry Clin Neurosci 1998;248(6):301–6.

[184] Brambilla P, Barale F, Soares JC. Perspectives on the use of anticonvulsants in the treatment of bipolar disorder. Int J Neuropsychopharmacol 2001;4(4):421–46.

[185] Brambilla P, Soares JC. The pharmacological treatment of acute mania. Psychiatr Clin North Am 2001;8:155–80.

[186] Hellweg R, Lang UE, Nagel M, et al. Subchronic treatment with lithium increases nerve growth factor content in distinct brain regions of adult rats. Mol Psychiatry 2002;7(6): 604–8.

[187] Jope RS. Anti-bipolar therapy: mechanism of action of lithium. Mol Psychiatry 1999;4(2): 117–28.

[188] Nonaka S, Katsube N, Chuang DM. Lithium protects rat cerebellar granule cells against apoptosis induced by anticonvulsants, phenytoin and carbamazepine. J Pharmacol Exp Ther 1998;286(1):539–47.

[189] Chen B, Wang JF, Hill BC, Young LT. Lithium and valproate differentially regulate brain regional expression of phosphorylated CREB and c-Fos [in process citation]. Brain Res Mol Brain Res 1999;70(1):45–53.

[190] Manji HK, Moore GJ, Chen G. Lithium up-regulates the cytoprotective protein Bcl-2 in the CNS in vivo: a role for neurotrophic and neuroprotective effects in manic depressive illness. J Clin Psychiatry 2000;61(Suppl 9):82–96.

[191] Wei H, Leeds PR, Qian Y, et al. Beta-amyloid peptide-induced death of PC 12 cells and cerebellar granule cell neurons is inhibited by long-term lithium treatment. Eur J Pharmacol 2000;392(3):117–23.

[192] Kirshenboim N, Plotkin B, Shlomo SB, et al. Lithium-mediated phosphorylation of glycogen synthase kinase-3b involves PI3 kinase-dependent activation of protein kinase C-alpha. J Mol Neurosci 2004;24(2):237–46.

[193] Moore GJ, Bebchuk JM, Hasanat K, et al. Lithium increases N-acetyl-aspartate in the human brain: in vivo evidence in support of bcl-2's neurotrophic effects? Biol Psychiatry 2000;48(1):1–8.

[194] Silverstone PH, Wu RH, O'Donnell T, et al. Chronic treatment with lithium, but not sodium valproate, increases cortical N-acetyl-aspartate concentrations in euthymic bipolar patients. Int Clin Psychopharmacol 2003;18(2):73–9.

[195] Moore GJ, Bebchuk JM, Wilds IB, et al. Lithium-induced increase in human brain grey matter. Lancet 2000;356(9237):1241–2.

[196] Sassi RB, Nicoletti M, Brambilla P, et al. Increased gray matter volume in lithium-treated bipolar disorder patients. Neurosci Lett 2002;329(2):243–5.

[197] Silverstone PH, Hanstock CC, Fabian J, et al. Chronic lithium does not alter human myo-inositol or phosphomonoester concentrations as measured by 1H and 31P MRS. Biol Psychiatry 1996;40(4):235–46.

[198] Silverstone PH, Rotzinger S, Pukhovsky A, et al. Effects of lithium and amphetamine on inositol metabolism in the human brain as measured by 1H and 31P MRS. Biol Psychiatry 1999;46(12):1634–41.

[199] Heuser IJ, Schweiger U, Gotthardt U, et al. Pituitary-adrenal-system regulation and psychopathology during amitriptyline treatment in elderly depressed patients and normal comparison subjects. Am J Psychiatry 1996;153(1):93–9.

[200] Soares JC, Mann JJ. The functional neuroanatomy of mood disorders. J Psychiatr Res 1997;31(4):393–432.

[201] Elliott R, Ogilvie A, Rubinsztein JS, et al. Abnormal ventral frontal response during performance of an affective go/no go task in patients with mania. Biol Psychiatry 2004; 55(12):1163–70.

[202] Lawrence NS, Williams AM, Surguladze S, et al. Subcortical and ventral prefrontal cortical neural responses to facial expressions distinguish patients with bipolar disorder and major depression. Biol Psychiatry 2004;55(6):578–87.

[203] Yurgelun-Todd DA, Gruber SA, Kanayama G, et al. fMRI during affect discrimination in bipolar affective disorder. Bipolar Disord 2000;2(3 Pt 2):237–48.

[204] Mitchell RL, Elliott R, Barry M, et al. Neural response to emotional prosody in schizophrenia and in bipolar affective disorder. Br J Psychiatry 2004;184:223–30.

[205] Chang K, Adleman NE, Dienes K, et al. Anomalous prefrontal-subcortical activation in familial pediatric bipolar disorder: a functional magnetic resonance imaging investigation. Arch Gen Psychiatry 2004;61(8):781–92.

[206] Malhi GS, Lagopoulos J, Ward PB, et al. Cognitive generation of affect in bipolar depression: an fMRI study. Eur J Neurosci 2004;19(3):741–54.

[207] Malhi GS, Lagopoulos J, Sachdev P, et al. Cognitive generation of affect in hypomania: an fMRI study. Bipolar Disord 2004;6(4):271–85.

[208] Curtis VA, Dixon TA, Morris RG, et al. Differential frontal activation in schizophrenia and bipolar illness during verbal fluency. J Affect Disord 2001;66(2–3):111–21.

[209] Blumberg HP, Leung HC, Skudlarski P, et al. A functional magnetic resonance imaging study of bipolar disorder: state- and trait-related dysfunction in ventral prefrontal cortices. Arch Gen Psychiatry 2003;60(6):601–9.

[210] Strakowski SM, Adler CM, Holland SK, et al. A preliminary fMRI study of sustained attention in euthymic, unmedicated bipolar disorder. Neuropsychopharmacology 2004; 29(9):1734–40.

[211] Blumberg HP, Martin A, Kaufman J, et al. Frontostriatal abnormalities in adolescents with bipolar disorder: preliminary observations from functional MRI. Am J Psychiatry 2003; 160(7):1345–7.

[212] Caligiuri MP, Brown GG, Meloy MJ, et al. An fMRI study of affective state and medication on cortical and subcortical brain regions during motor performance in bipolar disorder. Psychiatry Res 2003;123(3):171–82.

[213] Caligiuri MP, Brown GG, Meloy MJ, et al. A functional magnetic resonance imaging study of cortical asymmetry in bipolar disorder. Bipolar Disord 2004;6(3):183–96.

ELSEVIER
SAUNDERS

Psychiatr Clin N Am
28 (2005) 469–480

PSYCHIATRIC
CLINICS
OF NORTH AMERICA

Hypothalamic-pituitary-adrenal Axis and Bipolar Disorder

C. Daban, PhD[a], E. Vieta, MD, PhD[a],
P. Mackin, MB, BS, PhD, MRCPsych[b],*,
A.H. Young, MB, ChB, MPhil, PhD, FRCPsych[b,c]

[a]*Bipolar Disorders Program, Hospital Clinic, University of Barcelona, Barcelona, Spain*
[b]*University of Newcastle Upon Tyne, Newcastle Upon Tyne, NE1 7RU United Kingdom*
[c]*University of Barcelona, Gran Via Corts Catalanes, 585 08007 Barcelona, Spain*

The role of dysfunctional endocrine systems in the pathogenesis of mood disorders has been the focus of research for many decades. The complexity of endocrine systems and their interaction with neural networks frustrated early attempts to establish links between endocrinology and neuropsychiatry [1]. In the past 40 years, considerable advances have been made in the field of neuroendocrinology, highlighting the etiopathogenic significance of endocrine systems in mood disorders. More recently, the hypothalamic-pituitary-adrenal (HPA) axis has been the focus of research investigating the pathogenesis of bipolar disorder. Novel therapeutic approaches targeting the HPA axis have also evolved. This article focuses specifically on the role of the HPA axis in bipolar disorder.

Glucocorticoids

Glucocorticoids are hormones that are end products of the HPA axis and are central to the stress response. During the acute stress response, glucocorticoids induce short-term adaptive changes such as mobilizing energy reserves. They are also involved in long-term adaptive changes such as shaping and regulating a number of physiologic processes including immune responsiveness and activation of the sympathetic nervous system Overproduction of glucocorticoids is generally linked to significant disruption of

---
* Corresponding author. University of Newcastle Upon Tyne, Newcastle Upon Tyne, NE1 7RU United Kingdom.
 E-mail address: Paul.Mackin@newcastle.ac.uk (P. Mackin).

0193-953X/05/$ - see front matter © 2005 Elsevier Inc. All rights reserved.
doi:10.1016/j.psc.2005.01.005

cellular functioning, which in turn leads to widespread physiologic dysfunction.

The hypothalamic-pituitary-adrenal axis

The HPA axis, as it name indicates, is a feedback loop including the hypothalamus, pituitary, and adrenal glands, regulatory neural inputs, and a variety of releasing factors and hormones (Fig. 1).

During physical or psychological stress, the HPA axis is activated. The hypothalamus secretes two hormones, corticotropin-releasing hormone (CRH) and arginine vasopressin. CRH acts on the pituitary to stimulate adrenocorticotropic hormone (ACTH) release. ACTH reaches the adrenal cortex through the systemic circulation and interacts with receptors on adrenocortical cells stimulating the production and release of cortisol.

Cortisol is a glucocorticoid stress hormone that has a panoply of central and peripheral effects mediated by two intracellular specialized glucocorticoid receptor subtypes: the high-affinity type I receptor or mineralocorticoid receptor (MR), and the low-affinity type II receptor or glucocorticoid receptor (GR). The relative contribution of the two receptors (GR and MR) in the regulation of HPA activity is not yet clear. MRs have a high affinity

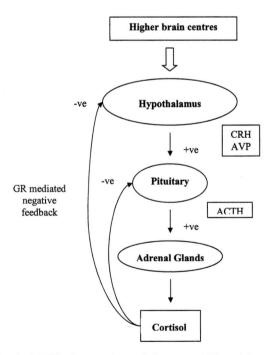

Fig. 1. The HPA axis. ACTH, adrenocorticotropic hormone; AVP, arginine vasopressin; CRH, corticotropin-releasing hormone; GR, glucocorticoid receptor; −ve, negative feedback; +ve, positive feedback.

for endogenous glucocorticoids, such as cortisol, and for the salt-regulating hormone aldosterone. The GRs have a relatively low affinity for cortisol but bind avidly to synthetic steroids such as dexamethasone (DEX). These differences in affinity suggest that MRs play an important role in regulating basal cortisol levels when hormone levels are low.

The HPA axis has an autoregulatory mechanism mediated by cortisol. When cortisol levels rise, as in response to stress or circadian fluctuations, the MRs are saturated. The GRs become the main transducer of glucocorticoid activity and, therefore, the primary mediator of the HPA feedback. The autoregulatory mechanisms are crucial in the maintenance of the homeostatic function of the HPA axis. Changes in GR number, function, or binding affinity may be important in altering the homeostatic function of the HPA axis observed in healthy individuals. The loop is completed with the negative feedback of cortisol on the pituitary, hypothalamus, and higher brain centers (Fig. 1).

HPA axis function is frequently investigated by measuring changes in cortisol, ACTH, or CRH release. The DEX suppression test (DST) is a sensitive measure of the functional integrity of the GR-mediated negative feedback mechanism: the cortisol-suppressing activity of the synthetic glucocorticoid, DEX, is an indicator of GR status [2]. A dose of DEX is given in the evening, and cortisol samples are obtained the next day. A normal response would be an inhibition of cortisol release resulting from negative feedback by DEX through the GRs. A newer test is the combined DEX/CRH challenge test, in which the HPA axis is both stimulated by the administration of CRH and inhibited with DEX [3]. This test is said to be more sensitive for detecting HPA abnormalities in patients with depression [3].

Cortisol and glucocorticoid receptor abnormalities in depression

In 1975, Stokes and colleagues [4] made the first observations of increased escape from cortisol suppression in patients with depression. Patients with HPA dysfunction, as in depressive disorder, respond with a paradoxically increased release of corticotropin and cortisol, whereas controls do not show such response. Many clinical studies have confirmed HPA hyperactivity in patients with severe mood disorders.

HPA hyperactivity is characterized by

- Hypersecretion of CRH
- Increased plasma cortisol levels
- Blunted corticotropin response to CRH
- Increased cortisol levels in the plasma, urine, and cerebrospinal fluid
- Exaggerated cortisol responses to corticotrophin
- Enlarged pituitary and adrenal glands

Some reports indicate that the chronic hypersecretion of cortisol could be caused by prolonged hypersecretion of CRH [5] and of ACTH [6]. Data regarding ACTH concentrations in depressed patients are inconsistent [7]. Some studies report higher ACTH levels [8], but others observe normal to low levels of ACTH in depressed patients [9,10]. One possible explanation is that the neurobiology of hypercortisolism changes over time during depressive episodes [7].

Successful treatment of depression is not always accompanied by a return to normal HPA axis function. Moreover, the recurrence of HPA abnormalities during remission of depressive symptoms is prognostically unfavorable and indicative of a relapse [11]. In another interesting study [12], remitted patients who relapsed with 6 months of discharge from inpatient treatment were those who had the higher ACTH and cortisol response to the DEX/CRH test; those who remained in stable remission did not differ in their responses, indicating that the DEX/CRH test may have prognostic significance. According to the authors, these elevated responses at discharge are biologic precursors of the relapse within a period of 6 months after discharge from hospital. An abnormal cortisol response in remitted patients could be a consequence of neuroadaptive changes that led to the depressive psychopathology and HPA dysregulation in the acute state [13]. Therefore, it seems that in the case of severe affective illnesses dysregulation of the HPA system can be considered as a putative neuroendocrine marker of these disorders.

Cortisol and bipolar disorder

Dysregulation of ACTH and cortisol response after CRH stimulation have been reported in bipolar patients, but altered states of the HPA axis have mostly been demonstrated in patients with depressive or mixed episodes [14–16]. This difference may arise from fewer studies of glucocorticoid regulation in patients with mania. Nevertheless, some interesting findings can be extracted from these studies. Reports of cortisol nonsuppression in response to DEX in both unipolar and bipolar disorders do suggest a primary GR abnormality in these disorders [17]. An enhanced response to corticotropin-releasing hormone was found in manic patients when compared with controls [18]. The differences disappeared when the patients who relapsed after 12 months were excluded. The changes in CRH secretion seem to appear before the manic or hypomanic symptoms are clinically evident. Therefore, this test seems to be trait-dependent. This enhanced response might result primarily from enhanced pituitary responsiveness to CRH.

Within the subtypes of affective illness, abnormal DST results are more common during depression in the course of bipolar disorder than in unipolar mood disorder [19–21]. HPA dysregulation does not seem to be linked to any particular type of episode, because these alterations were found in patients during acute depression and during mania [20]. Others postulate that HPA alterations are not state markers of bipolar disorder because circadian hypersecretion of cortisol occurred in depressed, hypomanic, and euthymic phases [22].

Pituitary gland volume, a marker of its functional status, has been used to examine HPA axis dysfunction [23]. A decreased volume of the pituitary was found persons with in bipolar disorder, when compared with healthy controls, but not in persons with unipolar disorder. This finding is consistent with pituitary hypoactivity in response to HPA stimulation in patients with bipolar disorder.

The severity of the manic episode seems to be highly correlated to the degree of neuroendocrine alteration. Anxiety, insomnia, and the intensity of depression were highly correlated with cortisol response [21]. Severity of depression was correlated with baseline cortisol concentration only in the bipolar group, not in the unipolar group. This finding may suggest a relationship between HPA pathology and severity of mood episode in bipolar disorder. A more heterogeneous status of the HPA system in unipolar patients might be related to greater diagnostic heterogeneity (and thus a lower validity of the phenotype).

Reports of cortisol function in mania are inconsistent. Some studies find normal cortisol suppression on the DST [24,25], but others find rates of nonsuppression comparable to those found in depression [26]. Moreover, it has been suggested that patients with mixed mania may be more likely than those with pure mania to exhibit DST nonsuppression. In Evans' study [25], patients with pure episodes of mania exhibited normal cortisol suppression, and the mixed-episode patients exhibited cortisol nonsuppression. Other studies have confirmed abnormal cortisol suppression in bipolar disorder, especially in mixed-episode patients [27,28].

Symptom resolution does not necessarily result in a normal response to the DEX/CRH test [20,21], indicating that HPA axis dysfunction may not simply be an epiphenomenon of illness. Bipolar patients exhibited significantly higher cortisol concentrations than unipolar patients in acute episodes as well as in remission, and the authors conclude that a higher degree of HPA system dysfunction is present in bipolar disorder than in unipolar depression [21]. In a pilot study, stable, lithium-responsive patients with bipolar disorder were found to have a significantly enhanced salivary cortisol response on waking, when compared with healthy controls [29]. This response is said to reflect an enduring tendency to abnormal cortisol regulation, even in stable patients. Higher cortisol concentrations were found in both nonremitted and remitted patients with bipolar disorder [30]. The HPA axis dysfunction could be a potential trait marker in bipolar disorder and thus possibly indicative of the core pathophysiologic process in this illness.

Abnormalities of the DEX/CRH test have been described in healthy subjects with a high familial risk for affective disorder [13]. The authors found increased cortisol secretion in the healthy group of probands, with levels intermediate between patients and controls. The type of parental affective disorder (unipolar or bipolar) was not relevant.

Recently Ellenboghen et al [31] described abnormalities in the HPA system of the young offspring of parents with bipolar disorder, suggesting that abnormalities in the HPA axis may precede the onset of affective disorders. Therefore, as in many other diseases, the development of the clinical phenotype of affective illness depends on environmental factors (family environment, life events, and stress, among others) as well as on genetic factors. Furthermore, these studies may lead to the discovery of candidate genes potentially involved in the transmission of affective illness.

The effect of treatments

An in vitro study has shown that some treatments used in mood disorders affect GR function [32]. Tricyclic antidepressants increase the GR mRNA in primary neuronal cultures, whereas in vivo studies show an increase in GR protein and binding capacity. These changes have also been reported, in rats, with the mood stabilizer lithium [33] and following electroconvulsive therapy [34]. According to some studies, lithium augmentation in treatment-resistant unipolar depression increases the cortisol response to the DEX/CRH test [35], but studies in bipolar disorder have found that lithium does not change cortisol response [30] or CRH concentrations [36].

Some studies have shown that the resolution of depressive symptoms with use of amitriptyline, paroxetine, or tianeptine normalizes the HPA axis [37–39]. According to Heuser et al [39], during antidepressant treatment, "a gradual reinstatement of appropriate glucocorticoid receptor function occurs," inducing normal responses to DEX/CRH. In another study, however, the absence of a treatment response to antidepressants did not alter cortisol output on the DEX/CRH test [40]. Furthermore, a significant correlation was found between carbamazepine dosage and cortisol response in the DEX/CRH test (cortisol response increases with increasing doses of carbamazepine) [12]. A more recent study has shown that patients taking carbamazepine had lower dexamethasone levels and were more likely to respond than those not taking carbamazepine [30]. When DEX windows were applied, however, there was no difference in DEX levels between patients and controls, suggesting that an effect of psychotropic medication on cortisol output through DEX metabolism is unlikely. Other studies have shown that neither citalopram [37] nor fluoxetine [38] has any effect on GR mRNA or GR binding, suggesting that selective serotonin reuptake inhibitors do not modulate GR expression or function.

Consequences of hypercortisolemia

Hypersecretion of CRH causing hypercortisolemia may be a result of impaired feedback mechanisms resulting from the GR abnormalities, such as decreased number or altered function. This view is supported by the demonstration of GR abnormalities in post-mortem studies of patients with severe mood disorders [41]. Animal studies have highlighted the importance of corticosteroids in influencing neurotransmitter receptor expression and function, long-term potentiation, and even cell survival. Manipulation of corticosteroids is likely, therefore, to influence the behavioral indices of neurotransmitter function, such as mood and cognition. Indeed, chronic administration of glucocorticoids impairs learning and memory in animals and humans [42], as well as causing marked atrophy of neurons in the hippocampal formation. It has been postulated that a similar neurodegenerative effect of cortisol may underlie some of the cognitive deficits observed in humans suffering from severe mood disorder [43]. Indeed, cortisol treatments induce cognitive deficits in healthy volunteers, deficits mediated in part by the frontal lobe, suggesting that this brain area may also be sensitive to the neurodegenerative effects of cortisol [44]. These deficits are reversible, but the cognitive deficits induced by hypercortisolism associated with mood disorder may not be reversible. High levels of cortisol may produce damage to the hippocampus, even after the acute episode has resolved. This hippocampal dysfunction, if present, could partially explain the impaired performance found in neuropsychologic measures of declarative learning and memory [45,46]. The hippocampus provides a negative feedback to the HPA and has an important role in declarative memory, emotional processing, and vulnerability to stress in patients with mood disorders [47].

Cognitive deficits do show some improvements on remission of affective symptoms (paralleling the return of normal HPA function), but this improvement is not sustained. Patients prospectively identified as euthymic still have deficits in executive control [48].

Cognitive deficits in bipolar disorder are associated with poor functional outcome [49]. A study that assessed cognitive functioning across different mood states in bipolar patients confirmed that even euthymic patients have cognitive deficits when compared with healthy controls. The number of previous manic episodes predicted cognitive dysfunction. Reports of higher ACTH and cortisol levels preceding manic episodes [16] further support the hypothesis that hypercortisolism leads to cognitive problems.

The argument that in mood disorders decreased GR function underlies excessive cortisol secretion and that a high cortisol level, in turn, induces deleterious effects on mood and cognition through an action on glucocorticoid receptors might seem contradictory. There are three possible explanations for the deleterious effects of high cortisol levels in the face of reduced GR function. (1) Elevated levels of cortisol may be sufficient to overcome the reduction in GR function and so produce an overall increase in effect. (2) It is possible that although GRs in the hippocampus and hypothalamus associated with autoregulation of the HPA axis are reduced in function, those in the other brain regions are normal. Thus, increased cortisol levels combined with normosensitive GRs might result in an increase in the deleterious effects of cortisol in some regions. (3) The deleterious effects of the high cortisol level may, at least in part, be mediated through MRs (or a change in the balance of activation of MRs and GRs) or through non–receptor-mediated events.

Therapeutic targets

The consequences HPA dysfunction described here may be central to the pathogenesis of affective disorders and cognitive deficits. Although clinical use of the currently available antiglucocorticoid drugs is limited by significant adverse side effect profiles, the development of drugs specifically targeting the glucocorticoid receptor may lead to innovative strategies in the treatment of mood disorders [50,51].

Corticotrophin-releasing hormone antagonists

Oversecretion of CRH resulting in hypercortisolism may be normalized by blockade of CRH receptors. Preclinical studies have suggested that CRH antagonists have clinical utility in conditions related to HPA hyperactivity, particularly anxiety disorders and depression. Clinical investigations of the use of CRH antagonists in a number of psychiatric disorders, including bipolar disorder, are currently underway.

Type II glucocorticoid receptor agonists

Activation of the GR-mediated negative-feedback mechanisms that regulate cortisol levels is another strategy for reducing circulating cortisol levels. The synthetic glucocorticoid DEX, given at doses of 3 to 4 mg for 4 days, has been shown to have antidepressant effects [52]. At this dose, DEX does not enter the central nervous system, and consequently central GRs are not activated. GRs at the level of pituitary are activated, leading to a lowering of endogenous circulating cortisol. The brief course of administration of DEX in these studies avoids the side effects associated with longer treatment.

Glucocorticoid receptor antagonists

Paradoxically, GR antagonists have also been advocated as agents with potential therapeutic properties for mood disorders. This therapy is based on the ability of the GR antagonist to block any detrimental effect of hypercortisolism and on the ability of an antagonist to increase the expression of its receptor. Administration of the GR antagonist results in an acute antiglucocorticoid effect while presumably causing a compensatory increase in GR number, leading to enhanced negative feedback on the HPA axis.

Several recent studies have increased the interest in the therapeutic efficacy of GR antagonists in the treatment of severe mood disorders. Initial clinical studies have examined the efficacy of the potent GR antagonist RU-486 (mifepristone). The results have been encouraging for major depression, but some clinical efficacy may have been masked by the prolonged administration of the drug (6 weeks) [53]. More recently, in a double-blind, placebo-controlled crossover study in five patients with psychotic depression, Belanoff and colleagues [54,55] found a rapid improvement in depression ratings and psychotic symptoms following only 4 days of treatment with mifepristone. These results have been replicated with a larger sample of patients. The results of the larger study suggest that high-dose treatment ($\geq$600 mg) for short periods (<7 days) is the optimal method of administration. The effects of other selective glucocorticoid receptor antagonists (ORG 34850, ORG 34116, ORG 34517) on the rat HPA were investigated. Chronic administration (1, 3, and 5 weeks) of GR antagonists resulted in only minor changes in brain GR levels, but each of them affected the HPA activity differently [56]. Once again, short-term administration seems preferable.

Animal studies suggest that the GR numbers are increased rapidly (within hours) after the administration of RU-486, which may restore feedback and thus reset the HPA axis. Such data also suggest that a brief period of treatment with the antagonist may be adequate for restoring normal HPA axis function. A short course of treatment might reduce the problems of noncompliance and side effects associated with longer-term administration.

The first preliminary double-blind, placebo-controlled, crossover study examining the effects of mifepristone (600 mg/day for 7 days) in 20 patients with bipolar disorder has been recently completed [57]. It was hypothesized that antiglucocorticoid treatments, particularly corticosteroid receptor antagonists, would improve neurocognitive functioning and depressive symptoms in bipolar disorder. Selective improvements were observed in neurocognitive functioning. Spatial memory, verbal fluency, and spatial recognition memory were significantly improved in patients treated with mifepristone compared with patients treated with placebo. Beneficial effects on mood were also found with a mean reduction of 5.1 points (28%) for the Hamilton Depression Rating Scale scores, and 6.05 points (26%) for the Montgomery-Asberg Depression Rating Scale scores, when compared with baseline. Similar improvements of mood or neurocognitive function were not observed in an identical trial of patients with schizophrenia [58]. These results require confirmation in studies of larger numbers of patients.

These data suggest that the GR antagonist RU-486 selectively improves neurocognitive function and may be antidepressant in bipolar disorder. In a recent study, RU-486 was the only one of the GR antagonists examined that increased both MR and GR binding in the frontal cortex [56]. This activity may explain the selective pattern of improvement in neurocognitive function seen in that study, which was restricted to tests that have been shown to be sensitive to frontal lobe dysfunction.

Summary

There is robust evidence demonstrating abnormalities of the HPA axis in bipolar disorder. Hypercortisolism may be central to the pathogenesis of depressive symptoms and cognitive deficits, which may in turn result from neurocytotoxic effects of raised cortisol levels. Manic episodes may be preceded by increased ACTH and cortisol levels, leading to cognitive problems and functional impairments. Identification and effective treatment of mood and cognitive symptoms of mood disorders are clinical goals, but currently available treatments may fall short of this ideal. Manipulation of the HPA axis has been shown to have therapeutic effects in preclinical and clinical studies, and recent data suggest that direct antagonism of GRs may be a future therapeutic strategy in the treatment of mood disorders.

Acknowledgments

The authors thank the Stanley Medical Research Institute for its generous support of their research programs.

References

[1] Michael RP, Gibbons JL. Interrelationships between the endocrine system and the neuropsychiatry. Int Rev Neurobiol 1963;5:243–302.

[2] Carroll BJ, Feinberg M, Greden JF, et al. A specific laboratory test for the diagnosis of melancholia: standardization, validation and clinical utility. Arch Gen Psychiatry 1981;38: 15–22.

[3] Heuser I, Yassouridis A, Holsboer F. The combined dexamethasone-CRH-test: a refined laboratory test for psychiatric disorder. J Psychiatry Res 1994;28:341–56.

[4] Stokes PE, Pick GR, Stoll PM, et al. Pituitary-adrenal function in depressed patients: resistance to dexamethasone suppression. J Psychiatry Res 1975;12:271–81.

[5] Nemeroff CB, Widerlov E, Bissette G, et al. Elevated concentrations of CSF corticotrophin-releasing factor-like immunoreactivity in depressed patients. Science 1984;226:1342–4.

[6] Reus VI, Joseph MS, Dallman MF. ACTH levels after the dexamethasone suppression in depression. N Engl J Med 1982;306:238–9.

[7] Parker KJ, Schatzberg AF, Lyons DM. Neuroendocrine aspects of hypercortisolism in major depression. Horm Behav 2003;43:60–6.

[8] Young EA, Carlson MS, Brown MB. Twenty-four-hour ACTH and cortisol pulsatility in depressed women. Neuropsychopharmacology 2001;25:267–76.

[9] Owens MJ, Nemeroff CB. The role of corticotropin releasing factor in the pathophysiology of affective and anxiety disorders: laboratory and clinical studies. Ciba Found Symp 1993; 172:296–308.

[10] Posener JA, De Battista C, Williams GH, et al. 24h monitoring of cortisol and corticotropin secretion in psychotic and non-psychotic major depression. Arch Gen Psychiatry 2000;57: 755–60.

[11] Holsboer F. The rationale for corticotropin-releasing hormone receptor (CRH-R) antagonists to treat depression and anxiety. J Psychiatr Res 1999;33:181–214.

[12] Zobel AW, Nickel T, Sonntag A, et al. Cortisol response in the combined dexamethasone/CRH test as predictor of relapse in patients with remitted depression: a prospective study. J Psychiatr Res 2001;35:83–94.

[13] Holsboer F, Lauer CJ, Schreiber W, et al. Altered hypothalamic pituitary adrenocortical regulation in healthy subjects at high family risk for affective disorders. Neuroendocrinology 1995;62:340–7.

[14] Gold PW, Chrousos G, Kellner C, et al. Psychiatric implications of basic and clinical studies with corticotropin-releasing factor. Am J Psychiatry 1984;141:619–27.

[15] Goodwin FK, Jamison KR. Manic-depressive illness. New York: Oxford University Press; 1990.

[16] Vieta E, Gasto C, Martinez de Osaba MJ, et al. Prediction of depressive relapse in remitted bipolar patients using corticotropin-releasing hormone challenge test. Acta Psychiatr Scand 1997;95:205–11.

[17] Zhou DF, Shen YC, Sch LN, et al. Dexamethasone suppression test and urinary MHPGX SO4 determination in depressive disorders. Biol Psychiatry 1987;22:883–91.

[18] Vieta E, Martinez-de-Osaba MJ, Colom F, et al. Enhanced corticotropin response to corticotropin-releasing hormone as a predictor of mania in euthymic bipolar patients. Psychol Med 1999;29:971–8.

[19] Rush AJ, Giles DE, Schlesser MA, et al. Dexamethasone response, thyrotropin-releasing hormone stimulation, rapid eye movement latency and subtypes of depression. Biol Psychiatry 1997;41:915–28.

[20] Schmider J, Lammers C, Gotthardt U, et al. Combined DEX/CRH test in acute and remitted manic patients, in acute depression and in normal controls. I. Biol Psychiatry 1995;38: 797–802.

[21] Rybakowski JK, Twardowska K. The dexamethasone/corticotropin-releasing hormone test in depression in bipolar and unipolar affective illness. J Psychiatr Res 1999;33:363–70.

[22] Cervantes P, Gelber S, Kin FN, et al. Circadian secretion of cortisol in bipolar disorder. J Psychiatry Neurosci 2001;26:411–6.

[23] Sassi R, Nicoletti M, Brambilla P, et al. Decreased pituitary volume in patients with bipolar disorder. Biol Psychiatry 2001;50:271–80.

[24] Schlesser MA, Winokur G, Sherman B. Hypothalamic-pituitary-adrenal axis activity in depressive illness. Arch Gen Psychiatry 1980;37:737–43.

[25] Evans DL, Nemeroff CB. The dexamethasone suppression test in mixed bipolar disorder. Am J Psychiatry 1983;140:615–7.

[26] Godwin CD, Greenberg LB, Shulka S. Consistent dexamethasone suppression test results with mania and depression in bipolar illness. Am J Psychiatry 1984;141:1263–5.

[27] Krishnan RR, Malbie AA, Davidson JRT. Abnormal cortisol suppression in bipolar patients with simultaneous manic and depressive symptoms. Am J Psychiatry 1983;140: 203–5.

[28] Swann AC, Strokes PE, Casper R, et al. Hypothalamic-pituitary-adrenocortical function in pure and mixed mania. Acta Psychiatr Scand 1992;85:2702–74.

[29] Deshauer D, Duffy A, Alda M, et al. The cortisol awakening response in bipolar illness: a pilot study. Can J Psychiatry 2003;48(7):462–6.

[30] Watson S, Gallagher P, Ritchie J, et al. Hypothalamic-pituitary-adrenal axis function in patients with bipolar disorder. Br J Psychiatry 2004;184:496–502.

[31] Ellenbogen MA, Hodgins S, Walker CD. High levels of cortisol among adolescent offspring of parents with bipolar disorder: a pilot study. Psychoneuroendocrinology 2004; 29:99–106.

[32] Pepin MC, Beaulieu S, Barrden N. Antidepressant regulate glucocorticoids receptor messenger RNA concentrations in primary neuronal cultures. Mol Brain Res 1989;6:77–83.

[33] Peiffer A, Veilleux S, Barden N. Antidepressant and other centrally acting drugs regulate glucocorticoid receptor messenger RNA levels in rat brain. Psychoneuroendocrinology 1991;16:505–15.

[34] Przegalinski E, Budziszewska B, Siwanowicz J, et al. The effect of repeated combined treatment with nifedipine and antidepressant drugs or electroconvulsive shock on the hippocampal corticosteroid receptors in rats. Neuropharmacology 1993;32:1397–400.

[35] Bschor T, Adli M, Baethge C, et al. Lithium augmentation increases the ACTH and cortisol response in the combined DEX/RH test in unipolar major depression. Neuropsychopharmacology 2002;27:470–8.

[36] Berrettini WH, Nurnemberg JI, Zerbe RL, et al. CSF neuropeptides in euthymic bipolar patients and controls. Br J Psychiatry 1987;150:208–12.

[37] Seckl JR, Fink G. Antidepressants increase glucocorticoid and mineralocorticoid receptor mRNA expression in rat in vivo. Neuroendocrinology 1992;55:621–6.

[38] Rossby SP, Nalpepa I, Huang M, et al. Norepinephrine-independent regulation of GRII mRNA in vivo by a tricyclic antidepressant. Brain Res 1995;687:79–82.

[39] Heuser I, Schweiger U, Gotthardt U, et al. Pituitary-adrenal-system regulation and psychopathology during amitriptyline treatment in elderly depressed patients and normal comparison subjects. Am J Psychiatry 1996;53:93–9.

[40] Kunzel HE, Binder EB, Nickel T, et al. Pharmacological and nonpharmacological factors influencing hypothalamic pituitary adrenocortical axis reactivity in acutely depressed psychiatric in-patients, measured by the DEX/CRH test. Neuropsychopharmacology 2003; 28:2169–78.

[41] Webster MJ, O'Grady JO, Orthman C, et al. Decreased glucocorticoid receptor mRNA levels in individuals with depression, bipolar disorder and schizophrenia. Schizophr Res 1999;41:111.

[42] Lupien SJ, McEwen BS. The acute effects of corticosteroids on cognition: integration of animal and human model studies. Brain Res Brain Res Rev 1997;24:1–27.

[43] Sapolsky RM, Krey LC, McEwen BS. The neuroendocrinology of stress and aging: the glucocorticoid cascade hypothesis. Endocrine Rev 1986;7:284–301.

[44] Young AH, Sahakian BJ, Robbins TW, et al. The effects of chronic administration of hydrocortisone on cognitive function in normal male volunteers. Psychopharmacology (Berl) 1999;145:260–6.

[45] Altshuler L. Bipolar disorder: are repeated episodes associated with neuroanatomic and cognitive changes? Biol Psychiatry 1993;33:563–5.

[46] Van Gorp WG, Altshuler L, Theberge D, et al. Cognitive impairment in euthymic bipolar patients with and without prior alcohol dependence. Arch Gen Psychiatry 1998;55:41–6.

[47] Brown ES, Rush AJ, McEwen BS. Hippocampal remodelling and damage by corticosteroids: implications for mood disorders. Neuropsychopharmacology 1999;21:474–84.

[48] Ferrier N, Stanton BR, Kelly TP, et al. Neuropsychological function in euthymic patients with bipolar disorder. Br J Psychiatry 1999;175:246–51.

[49] Martinez-Aran A, Vieta E, Colom F, et al. Cognitive impairment in euthymic bipolar patients: implications for clinical and functional outcome. Bipolar Disord 2004;6:1–9.

[50] Reus VI, Wolkowitz OM. Antiglucocorticoid drugs in the treatment of depression. Expert Opin Investig Drugs 2001;10:1789–96.

[51] Vieta E. Novedades en el tratamiento del trastorno bipolar. Madrid: Medica Panamericana; 2003.

[52] Arana GW, Santos AB, Laraia MT, et al. Dexamethasone for the treatment of depression: a randomized, placebo-controlled, double blind trial. Am J Psychiatry 1995;152:265–7.

[53] Murphy BE, Filipini D, Ghadirian AM. Possible use of glucocorticoid receptor antagonists in the treatment of major depression: preliminary results using RU-486. J Psychiatry Neurosci 1993;18:209–13.

[54] Belanoff JK, Flores BH, Kalezhan M, et al. Rapid reversal of psychotic depression using mifepristone. J Clin Psychopharmacol 2001;21:516–21.

[55] Belanoff JK, Rotschild AJ, Cassidy F, et al. An open label trial of C-1073 (mifepristone) for psychotic major depression. Biol Psychiatry 2002;52:386–92.

[56] Bachman CG, Linthorst AC, Holsboer F, et al. Effect of chronic administration of selective glucocorticoid receptor antagonists on the rat hypothalamo-pituitary-adrenocortical axis. Neuropsychopharmacology 2003;28:1056–67.

[57] Young AH, Gallagher P, Watson S, et al. Improvements in neurocognitive function and mood following adjunctive treatment with mifepristone (RU-486) in bipolar disorder. Neuropsychopharmacology 2004;29:1538–45.

[58] Gallagher P, Watson S, Smith M, et al. Efficacy of mifepristone (RU-486) in schizophrenia. Acta Psychiatr Scand 2004;110(Suppl):20.

ELSEVIER
SAUNDERS

Psychiatr Clin N Am
28 (2005) 481–498

PSYCHIATRIC
CLINICS
OF NORTH AMERICA

Recent Findings on the Genetic Basis of Bipolar Disorder

Jennifer L. Payne, MD*, James B. Potash, MD, MPH,
J. Raymond DePaulo, Jr, MD

*Department of Psychiatry and Behavioral Sciences, Johns Hopkins School of Medicine,
Baltimore, 600 North Wolfe Street, Meyer 3-181, Baltimore, MD 21287, USA*

Bipolar disorder has long been known to have a substantial genetic contribution. Compared with a 1% incidence rate in the general population, the incidence rate for first-degree relatives of a patient with bipolar disorder is about 7%, and a monozygotic twin of a bipolar patient has about a 60% likelihood of developing the illness [1–3]. What began as a search for a specific gene for bipolar disorder has now become a search for multiple susceptibility genes as it has become clear that the genetic basis of bipolar disorder probably involves multiple genes interacting with each other and with environmental components in as-yet mysterious ways. This article reviews the most recent findings and the emerging picture in the genetics of bipolar disorder.

Basic concepts and definitions

There are, in general, a series of logical steps to take when attempting to establish and understand the genetic basis for a trait or illness. The first is to establish familiality, that is, to determine if the trait or illness runs in families and may therefore have a genetic basis. The familiality of bipolar disorder is well established by family studies. The second step is to determine whether the familiality is based on a genetic relationship rather than an environmental one. The genetic relationship for bipolar disorder also is well established in many twin studies and a few adoption studies [3,4].

Once a genetic basis is established, the next logical step is to localize the genes that increase the risk for bipolar disorder. Linkage studies are

---

* Corresponding author.
E-mail address: jpayne5@jhmi.edu (J.L. Payne).

designed to identify a chromosomal region or regions that contain a susceptibility gene by using statistical techniques to measure the cosegregation of the phenotype (in this case bipolar disorder) and DNA markers distributed across all 23 human chromosomes [5,6]. A phenotype and markers on a chromosomal segment are said to be linked when they are transmitted together from affected parents to affected offspring more often than expected by chance. A logarithm of the odds (LOD) score is a statistical measure that estimates the probability that two genetic loci are linked. It measures the logarithm of the ratio of the odds favoring linkage to the odds against linkage. The value of the linkage statistic required to research statistical significance at the $P < 0.05$ level varies based on the number of markers and the number of phenotype definitions used. Schulze and McMahon [7] provide a more in-depth discussion of the statistical basis for the LOD score. In 1995 Lander and Kruglyak [8] established standards by which genetic linkage studies are judged for statistical significance. In general (depending upon the method used) a LOD score of 3.6 is considered statistically significant (ie, is statistically likely to occur 0.05 times in a genome scan by chance alone), whereas a score of 2.2 is considered suggestive, because values of this size will occur by chance alone only once per genome scan.

Genetic association studies are used to establish whether a particular form or variant of a gene is associated with a trait or disease and can either follow or complement linkage studies. Association studies are based on the common variations in genes known as single nucleotide polymorphisms (SNPs) in which a single nucleotide varies among individuals. SNPs occur approximately once in every 1000 base pairs of DNA [9]. Association studies compare the frequencies of particular alleles, or forms of a gene, between a group with a particular trait or illness and a control sample. Candidate genes are chosen based either on their function or position. Functional candidate genes are thought to have some biologic basis for a role in bipolar disorder, whereas positional candidates reside in regions that have previously been shown to have evidence for linkage in bipolar disorder and may or may not have a known biologic basis for a role in the development of bipolar disorder.

Linkage studies in bipolar disorder

Since the first genome-wide linkage scan in bipolar disorder was performed in 1993 [10], there have been multiple positive findings that have not been subsequently replicated. To date there have been 21 genome-wide linkage scans in bipolar disorder, with only six meeting criteria for significant linkage (Fig. 1). These regions are 8q24 [11,12], 15q14 [13], 18q12 [14], 21q23 [15,16], and 22q11-13 [17]. The study supporting 15q14 was for lithium-responsive family members only [13]. In addition, the study supporting 18q12 was done in families that were collected for both schizophrenia and bipolar disorder [14].

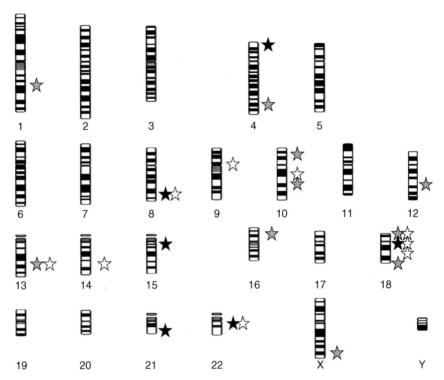

Fig. 1. Chromosomal regions implicated in bipolar disorder (based on individual studies and two meta-analyses).

Despite achieving genome-wide significance, however, these findings have not been consistently replicated by other studies. Regions that have been repeatedly implicated, although without achieving genome-wide significance, are 4p15 [18], 4q32-35 [19], 10q21-26 [20], 12q24 [21,22], 13q32 [23,24], 16p12-13 [20,25], 18p11 [26,27], 18q22-23 [28–30], and Xq24-28 [31,32]. The study by Detera-Wadleigh et al [23] that identified 13q32 as a potential locus for bipolar disorder just missed meeting criteria for significance with a LOD score of 3.5 and also found suggestive linkages on 4p16, 12q23-24, and 21q22. In addition, Shink et al [22] identified a suggestive region at 12q24 by genome-wide linkage with a LOD score of 3.35 that under a model-free analysis led to a significant LOD score of 5.05.

Meta-analyses

There have been two meta-analyses of linkage studies in bipolar disorder. The first, in 2002, included data from 11 genome scans [33]. This study found two regions of genome-wide significance, 13q32 and 22q12-13. The second meta-analysis [34] examined 18 genome scans but found no genome-wide significant linkage regions. Regions that had suggestive significance

($P < 0.01$) included 9p21-22, 10q11-22, and 14q24-32. Two of these regions (9p21-22 and 14q24-32) had not been highlighted by any prior study. The two candidate regions from the 2002 meta-analysis [33] were not statistically significant regions in this study. The differences between the results from the two meta-analyses are perhaps attributable to differences in the studies were included and how they were weighted.

One important conclusion from the multiple genome scans resulting in multiple linkage findings with few replications is that there is not a single major locus for bipolar disorder (ie, one that explains > 50% of the risk in > 50% of people with bipolar disorder) [35,36]. Instead, there are likely to be several susceptibility loci of smaller effect that increase the risk for developing the disorder in a non-Mendelian manner. Most bipolar genetics researchers have concluded that bipolar disorder is the result of the interaction between multiple genes and environmental factors. Several other reasons for the difficulty in identifying bipolar disorder loci are discussed in the next section.

Problems underlying the identification of linkage regions in bipolar disorder

One difficulty in linkage studies of bipolar disorder is the age of onset of the illness: although the onset is often in early adulthood, patients can develop the illness at any point during their lifetime. Thus, the identification of unaffected family members may be inaccurate in some families used as the basis for the linkage analysis. Schulze and McMahon [7] outline three other problems that underlie the difficulties in identifying linkage regions in bipolar disorder: locus heterogeneity, phenotype definition, and sample size.

Locus heterogeneity

Locus heterogeneity refers to the possibility that mutations in different genes can result in the same phenotype. A good example is Alzheimer's disease, in which clinically and neuropathologically similar cases have been found to have mutations in several different genes [37–39]. Locus heterogeneity results in a low likelihood of a successful linkage analysis, because different loci are involved in individual cases. Approaches to this problem include collecting data from genetically isolated populations, focusing on familial patterns of illness, and seeking families that are enriched for clinically severe phenotypes [7]. One criticism of bipolar genetic studies to date is that different studies have used different ascertainment schemes that may increase locus heterogeneity across samples [40].

Phenotype definition

Twin and family studies indicate that clinically distinct forms of affective disorders including major depression, bipolar I and II disorder, and schizoaffective disorder occur in the same families [4,41,42]. Major depression, for example, is also quite common in the general population; therefore, in a given family, a case of major depression may not have the same genetic basis as cases of bipolar disorder in other members of the family. Many studies in bipolar disorder therefore have not identified individuals with major depression as affected in the analysis or have defined the affected phenotype as narrowly as possible (eg, including only bipolar I individuals). Another approach to address this issue is to study endophenotypes (as discussed later), attempting to identify a subgroup of patients on a biologic basis. This approach has been useful in schizophrenia [43] and panic disorder [44]. Potentially useful endophenotypes in bipolar disorder include lithium responsiveness, the presence of white matter hyperintensities, and P300-evoked potentials (as discussed later).

Sample size

Perhaps the most straightforward problem underlying the lack of findings in linkage analysis in bipolar disorder is sample size. Risch and Merikangas [45] estimated that the sample sizes needed to detect a disease locus with a frequency of 50% and conferring a twofold increase in risk would require at a minimum 2500 affected sibling-pair families for linkage and 340 families for association studies. To date, no linkage study in bipolar disorder has achieved this goal, although there have been promising linkage findings despite this limitation. The National Institute of Mental Health (NIMH) Genetics Initiative Bipolar Collaborative has amassed the largest sample to date with more than 650 families, although an analysis of the full data set has not yet been completed. Meta-analyses may also be helpful in achieving the goal of larger sample sizes.

Association studies in bipolar disorder

There have been multiple association studies in bipolar disorder over the last 10 years. As described previously, association studies attempt to link variations in genes with a disease or illness. Many of the polymorphisms investigated are common variants in the population at large that, in the setting of other genetic factors or environmental factors, lead to the illness known as bipolar disorder. Thus, not all individuals with the risk polymorphism will develop the disease.

A number of methodologic issues plague many of these studies and probably contribute to nonreplication, as discussed previously. In many of these studies, the number of bipolar subjects is small, and most investigators have used gene variants that are not known to affect gene function. In addition, because there is little understanding of the underlying pathogenesis of bipolar disorder, the level of certainty about what constitutes a functional candidate gene is low.

The choice of control samples in association studies is another area where methodological problems may lead to false-positive results and subsequent nonreplication. Studies in which the control sample is drawn from unrelated individuals (either to each other or the control sample) suffer from false association caused by unknown population stratification (and therefore inadequate case-control sample matching). Family-based studies in which the control samples are drawn from relatives of the case sample circumvent this issue and therefore are less prone to false-positive results. Family-based approaches are, however, less statistically powerful than case-control studies and therefore are more prone to false-negative results [46].

Despite these limitations, there are a number of interesting candidate gene studies, which are discussed here. Each of these genes has had at least two positive association studies and few, if any, negative studies.

G72/G30

Two genes of unknown function, *G72* and *G30*, which overlap each other in the same stretch of DNA, have perhaps the strongest evidence for association with bipolar disorder. These genes were originally discovered as positional candidate genes in the 13q32 linkage region in schizophrenia [47]. *G72* activates D-amino acid oxidase, which in turn oxidizes D-serine, which activates *N*-methyl-D aspartate glutamate receptors. Four independent samples have demonstrated statistically significant associations between SNPs in or near this gene with bipolar disorder [48–50]. Because several schizophrenia samples have also demonstrated association with this gene, *G72/G30* may represent the first bipolar/schizophrenia overlap genes.

Brain-derived neurotrophic factor

Another exciting candidate gene is brain-derived neurotropic factor (BDNF). *BDNF* is an important member of the neurotrophin family and is known to affect neuronal outgrowth, differentiation, synaptic connectivity, and neuronal repair [51,52] for a broad range of neuronal cell types including serotonergic neurons [53]. Although the pathophysiology underlying depression and mood disorders in general is not understood fully, one proposal is that decreased *BDNF* expression is associated with depression in vulnerable individuals [54–56]. Serum *BDNF* levels were also recently shown to be significantly lower in patients with depression [57].

Two studies have associated the *BDNF* gene with bipolar disorder. Sklar et al [58] examined 76 candidate genes in 136 parent-proband (case) trios in a sample collected at Johns Hopkins and found that the *BDNF* gene was significantly associated with bipolar disorder. The association of bipolar disorder with the *BDNF* gene was then retested in an independent population of bipolar patients, and the results were consistent with the original finding. Neves-Pereira [59] showed that a particular polymorphism in the *BDNF* gene, a missense polymorphism, Val66Met, was preferentially transmitted to affected individuals, and analysis suggested that a DNA variant in the vicinity of the *BDNF* locus conferred susceptibility to bipolar disorder. In support of these findings, Sen et al [60] found a significant association between the Val66Met polymorphism and neuroticism, a personality trait associated with depression. These findings were not replicated in three Asian bipolar samples, however [61–63]. The failure to replicate the *BDNF* association in Asian populations may represent an ethnic difference in susceptibility genes. Nonetheless, the findings with the *BDNF* gene remain intriguing given its putative role in the brain and possibly in depression.

The serotonin transporter

As reviewed later, the serotonin transporter gene, *5-HTT*, has two different versions of the promoter region: short and long. The short version has been found to result in lower levels of gene expression than the long form. Four studies in bipolar disorder have shown a positive relationship between the short version and illness, but 12 other studies were negative [64–86]. Craddock et al [87] performed a meta-analysis of the 11 case-controlled studies (the other five were family based) and found no evidence for a significant effect. Two studies found an association with the short version and violent suicide attempts in bipolar disorder [88,89], however, and a third study found an association with completed suicide [90]. Rujescu et al [91], on the other hand, found no evidence for an association between the short variant and violent suicide in a sample of subjects who primarily had bipolar disorder.

There is some evidence that a second polymorphism in the *5-HTT* gene, a repeat in intron 2, influences gene expression in a transgenic mouse model [92]. There have been six positive studies and nine negative ones in bipolar disorder for this polymorphism [64–86].

Monoamine oxidase A

The monoamine oxidase A (*MAOA*) gene encodes an enzyme that breaks down the monoamine neurotransmitters including dopamine, norepinephrine, and serotonin. Given the clinical usefulness of MAO-inhibitor antidepressant medications, it is not surprising that this gene has been examined for association with recurrent depression and bipolar disorder. Twelve studies have examined four *MAOA* polymorphisms in bipolar disorder or bipolar disorder plus major depression [87–105]. Four have been positive, and nine have been negative. Two meta-analyses using the case-control method have been performed, one with pooled data from seven studies, the other with five studies [102,104]. Preisig et al [104] found that an allele in a microsatellite marker in intron 2 was 1.55 times more common in white bipolar cases than in controls, and a second variant in the same area was 2.65 times more common in Japanese bipolar subjects than in controls.

Catechol-O-methyltransferase

The catechol-O-methyltransferase gene codes for an enzyme that degrades dopamine and norepinephrine. It is located within 22q11 and has a functional SNP with a variant coding for methionine that has a three- to fourfold lower level of enzyme activity than the variant coding for valine. There have been five positive association studies for the methionine variant with bipolar disorder and seven negative ones [106–117]. A meta-analysis of seven case-control studies found a modest but statistically significant effect [87]. Three family-based studies were negative, however [111,115,116].

Future studies

The NIMH Genetics Initiative Bipolar Collaborative is in the process of ascertaining and assessing 5000 bipolar cases, which will provide a sample with ample power to detect genes with modest but real effects on bipolar susceptibility.

Clinical subtyping as an approach to the genetics of bipolar disorder

Evidence to date indicates that multiple genes of small effect are likely to be involved in the development of bipolar disorder. One approach to identifying these genes, called clinical subtyping, is to identify groups of subjects on a clinical basis who may be genetically similar. A related concept, endophenotype subtyping, identifies subgroups of patients on a biologic basis. Subtyping reduces genetic heterogeneity and ultimately increases the likelihood of finding the genetic risk factors for a genetically complex illness such as bipolar disorder. This approach has been used successfully in other complex disorders such as breast cancer and Alzheimer's disease. In both of these illnesses, families with early-onset illness were identified, and the genetic basis for the illness in these families was determined. This knowledge led to a greater understanding of the underlying biology in each of these illnesses and, in turn, has started to shed light on cases that are not familial or early onset.

Several clinical subtypes that show evidence of familiality in bipolar disorder include the presence of psychotic features, bipolar II disorder, comorbid panic and anxiety disorders, early onset of the illness, cognitive decline, rapid cycling, and comorbid attention deficit hyperactivity disorder. Endophenotypes that have been explored in bipolar disorder include lithium responsiveness, the presence of white matter hyperintensities, and P300-evoked potentials. Evidence for several of the subtypes that show promise and that have shown some evidence for linkage to a particular chromosomal area is described below.

Psychosis

Potash et al [118,119] found evidence for familial aggregation of psychotic symptoms in families with bipolar disorder in two separate samples. They found that if a proband with bipolar I disorder had psychotic symptoms, the odds that a relative with bipolar I also had psychotic symptoms were 3.17 ($P < 0.0039$). Potash et al [120] then tested the hypothesis that bipolar families in which multiple members had psychotic symptoms would show evidence of linkage to regions that previously had been implicated in both bipolar and schizophrenic pedigrees. These regions include 10p12-14, 18p11.2, 13q32, and 22q11-13 [121]. Ten of 65 families that had three or more members with psychotic mood disorder showed suggestive evidence of linkage to 13q31 and 22q12. The gene complex *G72/G30* is located on 13q33, not far from the 13q31 linkage peak, and, as discussed previously, four bipolar and five schizophrenia samples have shown statistically significant association with *G72/G30*.

Bipolar II disorder

Three studies have demonstrated familial aggregation of bipolar II disorder [122–124]. McMahon et al [29] demonstrated that a subgroup of 15 families (of 58 that were ascertained) that contained bipolar II sibling pairs demonstrated significant linkage with a LOD score of 4.67 to chromosome 18q21-22. Subsequent genotyping of more markers has increased the LOD score to 5.42 [125].

Comorbid panic and anxiety symptoms

MacKinnon et al [126,127] have demonstrated familial aggregation of comorbid panic disorder in families with bipolar disorder in two independent samples. MacKinnon then showed that families with bipolar disorder that contained at least one member affected with panic disorder demonstrated stronger linkage to chromosome 18 than did families without panic disorder [128].

Lithium responsiveness

Only a few small studies have investigated the familial aggregation of lithium responsiveness. The largest demonstrated a 67% response rate in family members of patients who responded to lithium, compared with 35% in relatives of patients who did not respond to lithium [129]. Turecki et al [13] conducted a genome scan in 31 families ascertained to be excellent lithium responders based on an average follow-up of 12 years. Significant evidence for linkage (LOD 3.46) was found on chromosome 15q14. Further analyses indicated that the locus on 15q was probably implicated in the etiology of bipolar disorder, whereas a suggestive locus on 7p11.2 was relevant for lithium response.

The role of environmental stress in affective illness

A new interest in gene–environment interaction has been spurred in part by an intriguing finding related to major depression. It is discussed here because it is the first study to demonstrate a proposition that has long been postulated: that life stress interacts with an underlying genetic vulnerability in the development of affective illness (in this case, major depression). Research of this kind may shed light on the path from genetic susceptibility to clinical manifestations of affective disorders, including bipolar illness.

Caspi et al [130] examined promoter region polymorphism in the serotonin transporter gene (5-HTT) in the setting of life stressors in such areas as relationships, employment, housing, health, and finances in a prospective-longitudinal study of a birth cohort. As noted earlier, the short promoter allele is associated with lower transcriptional efficiency than the long allele. Several studies have attempted to find an association between the short allele and the development of depression, but the results have been inconclusive [131]. Based on the possibility that the 5-HTT gene could modulate the serotonergic response to stress, the researchers examined the role of life stress in the development of depressive symptoms in individuals with one or two copies of the short allele. A significant association was found between the development of depression and suicidality in response to life events in individuals with either one or two copies of the short allele. In contrast, life stress did not predict the development of depressive symptoms in individuals with two copies of the long allele. Several attempts at replicating this work are ongoing, and further research using the gene–environment interaction paradigm is underway.

Summary and future directions

The genetic basis for bipolar disorder is complex and likely to be the cumulative effect of multiple genes of modest effect. The genetic basis for the illness may vary from family to family, and mutations or variations in different genes may lead to the same phenotype of mood disorder. Finally, the role of environmental influences in the development of bipolar disorder and how the environment interacts with genetic vulnerability is only beginning to be explored.

Linkage studies in bipolar disorder to date have been somewhat disappointing, in that statistically significant linkage has been identified in only a few regions, and most studies are not replicated. Studies now ongoing are working to rectify the problems associated with these results including ascertainment issues and sample size limitations. Clinical subtyping may help improve the power of linkage studies by defining more genetically homogeneous samples. Association studies in bipolar disorder are beginning to bear fruit. The identification of genes such as *G72/G30* and *BDNF* that seem to be associated with bipolar disorder in at least some samples is an important step forward. The ongoing collection of large samples of cases, for example through the NIMH Genetics Initiative, will provide the power needed to detect small gene effects and to study interactions between genes as well as between genes and the environment.

A vision for psychiatry and bipolar disorder

The identification of genes for bipolar disorder is an important goal for psychiatry. Benefits such as diagnostic testing and genotype-specific prognosis are important to patients. Prophylactic treatment for patients at high risk for the development of bipolar disorder is another potential benefit. Perhaps just as important, understanding the genetic basis for bipolar disorder is likely to lead to an understanding of the biologic basis for the illness and ultimately to improved treatments specifically designed to target the underlying pathophysiology.

During the next 15 to 30 years, two defining milestones for bipolar research will be the discovery of the pathogenic steps that lead to bipolar disorder and the formulation of accurate diagnostic tests and treatments that are more effective based on this knowledge. The recent progress in Alzheimer's disease, which can be related directly to genetic discoveries, suggests what is possible and indicates what expectations are reasonable. It is only a slight exaggeration to state that it is possible to give Alzheimer's disease to a mouse and to cure it. Creating a realistic model for bipolar disorder will be much more challenging because of the lack of molecular understanding of the pathogenesis of bipolar disorder and the fundamentally greater difficulty in measuring affective outcomes rather than cognitive ones. This goal will be attainable once the important genes that contribute to the risk for bipolar disorder are known and the rudiments of their function are understood. The time required for identifying the genes and their functional relationships even at the molecular level will be significant. Because existing treatments for bipolar disorder are relatively effective (and therefore are an indication of potential pathogenic mechanisms), moving forward from identification of the genes that increase the risk for bipolar disorder to an understanding of the pathogenesis of bipolar disorder may ultimately be a simpler task than in Alzheimer's disease. The work of discovery in the causal mechanisms of psychiatric disorders is multidisciplinary and will have great impact on the field. The development of new models of care derived from the discoveries about the pathogenesis of clinical psychiatric disorders will change fundamentally the way psychiatrists think about their patients and practice their specialty. Because the brain is the most complex organ, the scientific challenges inherent in this task cannot be underestimated. The harnessing of molecular neurobiology, neuropharmacology, imaging technology, and genetics makes radical dissection of psychiatric disorders an achievable goal.

References

[1] Goodwin FK, Jamison KR. Manic-depressive illness. New York: Oxford University Press; 1990. p. 938.

[2] Craddock N, Jones I. Genetics of bipolar disorder. J Med Genet 1999;36:585–94.

[3] Potash JB, DePaulo JR Jr. Searching high and low: a review of the genetics of bipolar disorder. Bipolar Disord 2000;2:8–26.

[4] Smoller JW, Finn CT. Family, twin and adoption studies of bipolar disorder. Am J Med Genet 2003;123C:48–58.

[5] Botstein D, White RL, Skolnick M, et al. Construction of a genetic linkage map in man using restriction fragment length polymorphisms. Am J Hum Genet 1980;32: 314–31.

[6] Weber JL, May PE. Abundant class of human DNA polymorphisms which can be typed using the polymerase chain reaction. Am J Hum Genet 1989;44:388–96.

[7] Schulze TG, McMahon FJ. Genetic linkage and association studies in bipolar affective disorder: a time for optimism. Am J Hum Genet 2003;123C:36–47.

[8] Lander E, Kruglyak L. Genetic dissection of complex traits: guidelines for interpreting and reporting linkage results. Nat Genet 1995;11:241–7.

[9] Venter JC, Adams MD, Myers EW, et al. The sequence of the human genome. Science 2001; 291:1304–51.

[10] Coon H, Jensen S, Hoff M, et al. A genome-wide search for genes predisposing to manic-depression, assuming autosomal dominant inheritance. Am J Hum Genet 1993;52(6): 1234–49.

[11] Cichon S, Schumacher J, Muller DJ, et al. A genome screen for genes predisposing to bipolar affective disorder detects a new susceptibility locus on 18q. Hum Mol Genet 2001; 10(25):2933–44.

[12] Avramopoulos D, Willour VL, Zandi PP, et al. Linkage of bipolar affective disorder on chromosome 8q24: follow-up and parametric analysis. Mol Psychiatry 2004;9:191–6.

[13] Turecki G, Grof P, Grof E, et al. Mapping susceptibility genes for bipolar disorder: a pharmacogenetic approach based on excellent response to lithium. Mol Psychiatry 2001; 6(5):570–8.

[14] Maziade M, Roy MA, Rouillard E, et al. A search for specific and common susceptibility loci for schizophrenia and bipolar disorder: a linkage study in 13 target chromosomes. Mol Psychiatry 2001;6(6):684–93.

[15] Straub RE, Lehner T, Luo Y, et al. A possible vulnerability locus for bipolar affective disorder on chromosome 21q22.3. Nat Genet 1994;8:291–6.

[16] Liu J, Juo SH, Terwilliger JD, et al. A follow-up linkage study supports evidence for a bipolar affective disorder locus on chromosome 21q22. Am J Med Genet 2001;105(2): 189–94.

[17] Kelsoe JR, Spence MA, Loetscher E, et al. A genome survey indicates a possible susceptibility locus for bipolar disorder on chromosome 22. Proc Natl Acad Sci U S A 2001; 98(2):585–90.

[18] Blackwood DH, He L, Morris SW, et al. A locus for bipolar affective disorder on chromosome 4p. Nat Genet 1996;12:427–30.

[19] Adams LJ, Mitchell PB, Fielder SL, et al. A susceptibility locus for bipolar affective disorder on chromosome 4q35. Am J Hum Genet 1998;62:1084–91.

[20] McInnis MG, Dick DM, Willour VL, et al. Genome-wide scan and conditional analysis in bipolar disorder: evidence for genomic interaction in the National Institute of Mental Health Genetics Initiative bipolar pedigrees. Biol Psychiatry 2003;54:1265–73.

[21] Morissette J, Villeneuve A, Bordeleau L, et al. Genome-wide search for linkage of bipolar affective disorders in a very large pedigree derived from a homogeneous population in Quebec points to a locus of major effect on chromosome 12q23-q24. Am J Med Genet 1999; 88:567–87.

[22] Shink E, Morissette J, Sherrington R, Barden N. A genome-wide scan points to a susceptibility locus for bipolar disorder on chromosome 12. Mol Psychiatry 2004 Oct 19; [Epub ahead of print].

[23] Detera-Wadleigh SD, Badner JA, et al. A high-density genome scan detects evidence for a bipolar-disorder susceptibility locus on 13q32 and other potential loci on 1q32 and 18p11.2. Proc Natl Acad Sci U S A 1999;96:5604–9.

[24] Liu C, Badner JA, Christian SL, et al. Fine mapping supports previous linkage evidence for a bipolar disorder susceptibility locus on 13q32. Am J Med Genet 2001;105:375–80.

[25] Edenberg HJ, Foroud T, Conneally M, et al. Initial genomic scan of the NIMH Genetics Initiative bipolar pedigrees: chromosomes 3, 5, 15, 16, 17 and 22. Am J Med Genet 1997;74: 238–46.

[26] Berrettini WH, Ferraro TN, Goldin LR, et al. Chromosome 18 DNA markers and manic-depressive illness: evidence for a susceptibility gene. Proc Natl Acad Sci U S A 1994;91: 5918–21.

[27] Schwab SG, Hallmayer J, Lerer B, et al. Support for a chromosome 18p locus conferring susceptibility to functional psychoses in families with schizophrenia, by association and linkage analysis. Am J Hum Genet 1998;63:1139–52.

[28] Stine OC, Xu J, Koskela R, et al. Evidence for linkage of bipolar disorder to chromosome 18 with parent-of-origin effect. Am J Hum Genet 1995;57:1384–94.

[29] McMahon FJ, Hopkins PJ, Xu J, et al. Linkage of bipolar affective disorder to chromosome 18 markers in a new pedigree series. Am J Hum Genet 1997;61:1397–404.

[30] Bennett P, Segurado R, Jones I, et al. The Wellcome trust UK-Iris bipolar affective disorder sibling-pair genome screen: first stage report. Mol Psychiatry 2002;7:189–200.

[31] Pekkarinen P, Terwilliger J, Bredbacka PE, et al. Evidence of a predisposing locus to bipolar disorder on Xq24-q27.1 in an extended Finnish pedigree. Genome Res 1995;5: 105–15.

[32] Stine OC, McMahon FJ, Chen L, et al. Initial genome screen for bipolar disorder in the NIMH genetics initiative pedigrees: chromosomes 2,11,13,14, and X. Am J Med Genet 1997;74:263–9.

[33] Badner JA, Gershon ES. Meta-analysis of whole-genome linkage scans of bipolar disorder and schizophrenia. Mol Psychiatry 2002;7(4):405–11.

[34] Sequardo R, Detera-Wadleigh SD, Levinson DF, et al. Genome scan meta-analysis of schizophrenia and bipolar disorder, part III: bipolar disorder. Am J Hum Genet 2003;73: 49–62.

[35] DePaulo JR. Genetics of bipolar disorder: where do we stand? Am J Psychiatry 2004;161: 595–7.

[36] Berrettini W. Genetics of major mood disorders. Psychiatry 2004;1(2):38–48.

[37] Burke JR, Roses AD. Genetics of Alzheimer's disease. Int J Neurol 1991;25:41–51.

[38] Goate A, Chartier-Harlin MC, Mullan M, et al. Segregation of a missense mutation in the amyloid precursor protein gene with familial Alzheimer's disease. Nature 1991;349: 704–6.

[39] Martin ER, Scott WK, Nance MA, et al. Association of single-nucleotide polymorphisms of the tau gene with late-onset Parkinson disease. JAMA 2001;286:2245–50.

[40] Prathikanti S, McMahon FJ. Genome scans for susceptibility genes in bipolar affective disorder. Ann Med 2001;33:257–62.

[41] Bertelsen A, Harvald B, Hauge M. A Danish twin study of manic depressive disorders. Br J Psychiatry 1977;130:330–51.

[42] Gershon ES, Hamovit J, Guroff JJ, et al. A family study of schizoaffective, bipolar I, bipolar II, unipolar, and normal control probands. Arch Gen Psychiatry 1982;39:1157–67.

[43] Adler LE, Pachtman E, Franks RD, et al. Neurophysiological evidence for a defect in neuronal mechanisms involved in sensory gating in schizophrenia. Biol Psychiatry 1982;17: 639–54.

[44] Gorman JM, Goetz RR, Dillon D, et al. Sodium D-lactate infusion of panic disorder patients. Neuropsychopharmacology 1990;3:181–9.

[45] Risch N, Merikangas K. The future of genetic studies of complex human diseases. Science 1996;273:1516–7.

[46] Risch N. Searching for genes in complex diseases: lessons from systemic lupus erythematosus. J Clin Invest 2000;105:1503–6.

[47] Chumakov I, Blumenfeld M, Guerassimenko O, et al. Genetic and physiological data implicating the new human gene G72 and the gene for D-amino acid oxidase in schizophrenia. Proc Natl Acad Sci U S A 2002;99(21):13675–80.

[48] Hattori E, Liu C, Badner JA, et al. Polymorphisms at the G72/G30 gene locus, on 13q33, are associated with bipolar disorder in two independent pedigree series. Am J Hum Genet 2003;72(5):1131–40.

[49] Chen YS, Akula N, Detera-Wadleigh SD, et al. Findings in an independent sample support an association between bipolar affective disorder and the G72/G30 locus on chromosome 13q33. Mol Psychiatry 2004;9:87–92.

[50] Schumacher J, Abon Jamra R, Frudenberg J, et al. Examination of G72 and D-amino-acid oxidase as genetic risk factors for schizophrenia and bipolar affective disorder. Mol Psychiatry 2004;9:203–7.

[51] Lindsay RM, Wiegrand SJ, Altar CA, et al. Neurotrophic factors: from molecule to man. Trends Neurosci 1994;17:182–90.

[52] Lewin GR, Barde YA. Physiology of neurotrophins. Annu Rev Neurosci 1996;19:289–317.

[53] Mamounas LA, Blue ME, Siuciak JA, et al. Brain-derived neurotrophic factor promotes the survival and sprouting of serotonergic axons in the mouse brain. J Neurosci 1995;15: 7929–39.

[54] Duman RS, Heninger GR, Nestler EJ. A molecular and cellular theory of depression. Arch Gen Psychiatry 1997;54:597–606.

[55] Altar CA. Neurotrophins and depression. Trends Pharmacol Sci 1999;20:59–61.

[56] Shelton RC. Cellular mechanisms in the vulnerability to depression response to antidepressants. Psychiatr Clin North Am 2000;23:713–29.

[57] Karege F, Perret G, Bondolfi G, et al. Decreased serum brain-derived neurotrophic factor levels in major depressed patients. Psychiatry Res 2002;109:143–8.

[58] Sklar P, Gabriel SB, McInnis MG, et al. Family-based association study of 76 candidate genes in bipolar disorder: BDNF is a potential risk locus. Brain-derived neurotrophic factor. Mol Psychiatry 2002;7(6):579–93.

[59] Neves-Pereira M, Mundo E, Muglia P, et al. The brain-derived neurotrophic factor gene confers susceptibility to bipolar disorder: evidence from a family-based association study. Am J Hum Genet 2002;71(3):651–5.

[60] Sen S, Nesse RM, Stoltenberg SF, et al. A BDNF coding variant is associated with the NEO personality inventory domain neuroticism, a risk factor for depression. Neuro-psychopharmacology 2003;28(2):397–401.

[61] Hong CJ, Huo SJ, Yen FC, et al. Association study of a brain-derived neurotrophic factor genetic polymorphism and mood disorders, age of onset and suicidal behavior. Neuopsychobiology 2003;48:186–9.

[62] Nakata K, Ujike H, Sakai A, et al. Association study of the brain-derived neurotrophic factor (BDNF) gene with bipolar disorder. Neurosci Lett 2003;337(1):17–20.

[63] Kunugi H, Iijima Y, Tatsumi M, et al. No association between the Val66Met polymorphism of the brain-derived neurotrophic factor gene and bipolar disorder in a Japanese population: a multicenter study. Biol Psychiatry 2004;56:376–8.

[64] Collier DA, Arranz MJ, Sham P, et al. The serotonin transporter is a potential susceptibility factor for bipolar affective disorder. Neuroreport 1996;7(10):1675–9.

[65] Collier DA, Stober G, Li T, et al. A novel functional polymorphism within the promoter of the serotonin transporter gene: possible role in susceptibility to affective disorders. Mol Psychiatry 1996;1(6):453–60.

[66] Battersby S, Ogilvie AD, Smith CA, et al. Structure of a variable number tandem repeat of the serotonin transporter gene and association with affective disorder. Psychiatr Genet 1996;6(4):177–81.

[67] Rees M, Norton N, Jones I, et al. Association studies of bipolar disorder at the human serotonin transporter gene (hSERT; 5HTT). Mol Psychiatry 1997;2(5):398–402.

[68] Oruc L, Verheyen GR, Furac I, et al. Association analysis of the 5–HT2C receptor and 5-HT transporter genes in bipolar disorder. Am J Med Genet 1997;74(5):504–6.

[69] Kunugi H, Hattori M, Kato T, et al. Serotonin transporter gene polymorphisms: ethnic difference and possible association with bipolar affective disorder. Mol Psychiatry 1997; 2(6):457–62.

[70] Bellivier F, Henry C, Szoke A, et al. Serotonin transporter gene polymorphisms in patients with unipolar or bipolar depression. Neurosci Lett 1998;255(3):143–6.

[71] Vincent JB, Masellis M, Lawrence J. Genetic association analysis of serotonin system genes in bipolar affective disorder. Am J Psychiatry 1999;156(1):136–8.

[72] Furlong RA, Ho L, Walsh C, et al. Analysis and meta-analysis of two serotonin transporter gene polymorphisms in bipolar and unipolar affective disorders. Am J Med Genet 1998; 81(1):58–63.

[73] Esterling LE, Yoshikawa T, Turner G, et al. Serotonin transporter (5-HTT) gene and bipolar affective disorder. Am J Med Genet 1998;81(1):37–40.

[74] Hoehe MR, Wendel B, Grunewald I, et al. Serotonin transporter (5-HTT) gene polymorphisms are not associated with susceptibility to mood disorders. Am J Med Genet 1998; 81(1):1–3.

[75] Mendes de Oliveira JR, Otto PA, Vallada H, et al. Analysis of a novel functional polymorphism within the promoter region of the serotonin transporter gene (5-HTT) in Brazilian patients affected by bipolar disorder and schizophrenia. Am J Med Genet 1998;81(3):225–7.

[76] Gutierrez B, Arranz MJ, Collier DA, et al. Serotonin transporter gene and risk for bipolar affective disorder: an association study in Spanish population. Biol Psychiatry 1998;43(11): 843–7.

[77] Kirov G, Rees M, Jones I, et al. Bipolar disorder and the serotonin transporter gene: a family-based association study. Psychol Med 1999;29(5):1249–54.

[78] Liu W, Gu N, Feng G, et al. Tentative association of the serotonin transporter with schizophrenia and unipolar depression but not with bipolar disorder in Han Chinese. Pharmacogenetics 1999;9(4):491–5.

[79] Bocchetta A, Piccardi MP, Palmas MA, et al. Family-based association study between bipolar disorder and DRD2, DRD4, DAT, and SERT in Sardinia. Am J Med Genet 1999; 88(5):522–6.

[80] Mynett-Johnson L, Kealey C, Claffey E, et al. Multimarker haplotypes within the serotonin transporter gene suggest evidence of an association with bipolar disorder. Am J Med Genet 2000;96(6):845–9.

[81] Saleem Q, Ganesh S, Vijaykumar M, et al. Association analysis of 5HT transporter gene in bipolar disorder in the Indian population. Am J Med Genet 2000;96(2):170–2.

[82] Mundo E, Walker M, Tims H, et al. Lack of linkage disequilibrium between serotonin transporter protein gene (SLC6A4) and bipolar disorder. Am J Med Genet 2000;96(3): 379–83.

[83] Ospina-Duque J, Duque C, et al. An association study of bipolar mood disorder (type I) with the 5-HTTLPR serotonin transporter polymorphism in a human population isolate from Colombia. Neurosci Lett 2000;292(3):199–202.

[84] Serretti A, Cristina S, Lilli R, et al. Family-based association study of 5-HTTLPR, TPH, MAO-A, and DRD4 polymorphisms in mood disorders. Am J Med Genet 2002;114(4): 361–9.

[85] Rotondo A, Mazzanti C, Dell'Osso L, et al. Catechol O-methyltransferase, serotonin transporter, and tryptophan hydroxylase gene polymorphisms in bipolar disorder patients with and without comorbid panic disorder. Am J Psychiatry 2002;159(1):23–9.

[86] Dimitrova A, Georgieva L, Nikolov I, et al. Major psychiatric disorders and the serotonin transporter gene (SLC6A4): family-based association studies. Psychiatr Genet 2002;12(3): 137–41.

[87] Craddock N, Dave S, Greening J. Association studies of bipolar disorder. Bipolar Disord 2001;3(6):284–98.

[88] Bellivier F, Szoke A, Henry C, et al. Possible association between serotonin transporter gene polymorphism and violent suicidal behavior in mood disorders. Biol Psychiatry 2000; 48(4):319–22.

[89] Courtet P, Baud P, Abbar M, et al. Association between violent suicidal behavior and the low activity allele of the serotonin transporter gene. Mol Psychiatry 2001;6(3):338–41.

[90] Bondy B, Erfurth A, de Jonge S, et al. Possible association of the short allele of the serotonin transporter promoter gene polymorphism (5-HTTLPR) with violent suicide. Mol Psychiatry 2000;5(2):193–5.

[91] Rujescu D, Giegling I, Sato T, et al. A polymorphism in the promoter of the serotonin transporter gene is not associated with suicidal behavior. Psychiatr Genet 2001;11(3): 169–72.

[92] MacKenzie A, Quinn J. A serotonin transporter gene intron 2 polymorphic region, correlated with affective disorders, has allele-dependent differential enhancer-like properties in the mouse embryo. Proc Natl Acad Sci U S A 1999;96(26):15251–5.

[93] Lim LC, Powell J, Sham P, et al. Evidence for a genetic association between alleles of monoamine oxidase A gene and bipolar affective disorder. Am J Med Genet 1995;60(4): 325–31.

[94] Kawada Y, Hattori M, Dai XY, et al. Possible association between monoamine oxidase A gene and bipolar affective disorder. Am J Hum Genet 1995;56(1):335–6.

[95] Craddock N, Daniels J, Roberts E, et al. No evidence for allelic association between bipolar disorder and monoamine oxidase A gene polymorphisms. Am J Med Genet 1995;60(4): 322–4.

[96] Nothen MM, Eggermann K, Albus M, et al. Association analysis of the monoamine oxidase A gene in bipolar affective disorder by using family-based internal controls. Am J Hum Genet 1995;57(4):975–8.

[97] Rubinsztein DC, Leggo J, Goodburn S, et al. Genetic association between monoamine oxidase A microsatellite and RFLP alleles and bipolar affective disorder: analysis and meta-analysis. Hum Mol Genet 1996;5(6):779–82.

[98] Muramatsu T, Matsushita S, Kanba S, et al. Monoamine oxidase genes polymorphisms and mood disorder. Am J Med Genet 1997;74(5):494–6.

[99] Parsian A, Todd RD. Genetic association between monoamine oxidase and manic-depressive illness: comparison of relative risk and haplotype relative risk data. Am J Med Genet 1997;74(5):475–9.

[100] Turecki G, Grof P, Cavazzoni P, et al. MAOA: association and linkage studies with lithium responsive bipolar disorder. Psychiatr Genet 1999;9(1):13–6.

[101] Kunugi H, Ishida S, Kato T, et al. A functional polymorphism in the promoter region of monoamine oxidase-A gene and mood disorders. Mol Psychiatry 1999;4(4):393–5.

[102] Furlong RA, Ho L, Rubinsztein JS, et al. Analysis of the monoamine oxidase A (MAOA) gene in bipolar affective disorder by association studies, meta-analyses, and sequencing of the promoter. Am J Med Genet 1999;88(4):398–406.

[103] Kirov G, Norton N, Jones I, et al. A functional polymorphism in the promoter of monoamine oxidase A gene and bipolar affective disorder. Int J Neuropsychopharmcol 1999;2(4): 293–8.

[104] Preisig M, Bellivier F, Fenton BT, et al. Association between bipolar disorder and monoamine oxidase A gene polymorphisms: results of a multicenter study. Am J Psychiatry 2000;157(6):948–55.

[105] Syagailo YV, Stober G, Grassle M, et al. Association analysis of the functional monoamine oxidase A gene promoter polymorphism in psychiatric disorders. Am J Med Genet 2001; 105(2):168–71.

[106] Biomed European Bipolar Collaborative Group. No association between bipolar disorder and alleles at a functional polymorphism in the COMT gene. Br J Psychiatry 1997;170: 526–8.

[107] Li T, Vallada H, Curtis D, et al. Catechol-O-methyltransferase Val158Met polymorphism: frequency analysis in Han Chinese subjects and allelic association of the low activity allele with bipolar affective disorder. Pharmacogenetics 1997;7(5):349–53.

[108] Gutierrez B, Bertranpetit J, Guillamat R, et al. Association analysis of the catechol O-methyltransferase gene and bipolar affective disorder. Am J Psychiatry 1997;154(1):113–5.

[109] Kunugi H, Vallada HP, Hoda F, et al. No evidence for an association of affective disorders with high- or low-activity allele of catechol-O-methyltransferase gene. Biol Psychiatry 1997; 42(4):282–5.

[110] Lachman HM, Kelsoe J, Moreno L, et al. Lack of association of catechol-O-methyltransferase (COMT) functional polymorphism in bipolar affective disorder. Psychiatr Genet 1997;7(1):13–7.

[111] Mynett-Johnson LA, Murphy VE, Claffey E, et al. Preliminary evidence of an association between bipolar disorder in females and the catechol-O-methyltransferase gene. Psychiatr Genet 1998;8(4):221–5.

[112] Papolos DF, Veit S, Faedda GL, et al. Ultra-ultra rapid cycling bipolar disorder is associated with the low activity catecholamine-O-methyltransferase allele. Mol Psychiatry 1998;3(4):346–9.

[113] Ohara K, Nagai M, Suzuki Y. Low activity allele of catechol-O-methyltransferase gene and Japanese unipolar depression. Neuroreport 1998;9(7):1305–8.

[114] Kirov G, Murphy KC, Arranz MJ, et al. Low activity allele of catechol-O-methyltransferase gene associated with rapid cycling bipolar disorder. Mol Psychiatry 1998;3(4):342–5.

[115] Kirov G, Jones I, McCandless F, et al. Family-based association studies of bipolar disorder with candidate genes involved in dopamine neurotransmission: DBH, DAT1, COMT, DRD2, DRD3 and DRD5. Mol Psychiatry 1999;4(6):558–65.

[116] Geller B, Cook EH Jr. Ultradian rapid cycling in prepubertal and early adolescent bipolarity is not in transmission disequilibrium with Val/Met COMT alleles. Biol Psychiatry 2000;47(7):605–9.

[117] Rotondo A, Mazzanti C, Dell'Osso L, et al. Catechol O-methyltransferase, serotonin transporter, and tryptophan hydroxylase gene polymorphisms in bipolar disorder patients with and without comorbid panic disorder. Am J Psychiatry 2002;159(1):23–9.

[118] Potash JB, Willour VL, Chiu YF, et al. The familial aggregation of psychotic symptoms in bipolar disorder pedigrees. Am J Psychiatry 2001;158(8):1258–64.

[119] Potash JB, Chiu YF, MacKinnon DF, et al. Familial aggregation of psychotic symptoms in a replication set of 69 bipolar disorder pedigrees. Am J Med Genet 2003;116:90–7.

[120] Potash JB, Zandi PP, Willour VL, et al. Suggestive linkage to chromosomal regions 13q31 and 22q12 in families with psychotic bipolar disorder. Am J Psychiatry 2003;160(4): 680–6.

[121] Berrettini WH. Are schizophrenic and bipolar disorders related? A review of family and molecular studies. Biol Psychiatry 2000;48(6):531–8.

[122] Gershon ES, Hamovit J, Guroff JJ, et al. A family study of schizoaffective, bipolar I, bipolar II, unipolar, and normal control probands. Arch Gen Psychiatry 1982;39(10): 1157–67.

[123] Andreasen NC, Rice J, Endicott J, et al. Familial rates of affective disorder. A report from the national Institute of Mental Health Collaborative Study. Arch Gen Psychiatry 1988;44: 461–9.

[124] Heun R, Maier W. Bipolar II disorders in six first-degree relatives. Biol Psychiatry 1993;34: 274–6.

[125] Schulze TG, Chen YS, Badner JA, et al. Additional, physically ordered markers increase linkage signal for bipolar disorder on chromosome 18q22. Biol Psychiatry 2003;53(3): 239–43.

[126] MacKinnon DF, McMahon FJ, Simpson SG, et al. Panic disorder with familial bipolar disorder. Biol Psychiatry 1997;42:90–5.

[127] MacKinnon DF, Zandi PP, Cooper J, et al. Comorbid bipolar disorder and panic disorder in families with a high prevalence of bipolar disorder. Am J Psychiatry 2002;159:30–5.

[128] MacKinnon DF, Xu J, McMahon FJ, et al. Bipolar disorder and panic disorder in families: an analysis of chromosome 18 data. Am J Psychiatry 1998;155:829–31.

[129] Grof P, Duffy A, Cavazzoni P, et al. Is response to prophylactic lithium a familial trait? J Clin Psychiatry 2002;63(10):942–7.

[130] Caspi A, Sugden K, Moffitt TE, et al. Influence of life stress on depression: moderation by a polymorphism in the 5-HTT gene. Science 2003;301:386–9.

[131] Lesch KP. Animal models of anxiety. In: Plomin R, DeFries JC, Craig IW, et al, editors. Behavioral genetics in the postgenomics era. Washington (DC): American Psychiatric Association; 2003. p. 389–424.

ELSEVIER SAUNDERS

Psychiatr Clin N Am
28 (2005) 499–505

PSYCHIATRIC CLINICS OF NORTH AMERICA

Index

Note: Page numbers of article titles are in **boldface** type.

Changing Your Address?

Make sure your subscription changes too! When you notify us of your new address, you can help make our job easier by including an exact copy of your Clinics label number with your old address (see illustration below.) This number identifies you to our computer system and will speed the processing of your address change. Please be sure this label number accompanies your old address and your corrected address—you can send an old Clinics label with your number on it or just copy it exactly and send it to the address listed below.

We appreciate your help in our attempt to give you continuous coverage. Thank you.

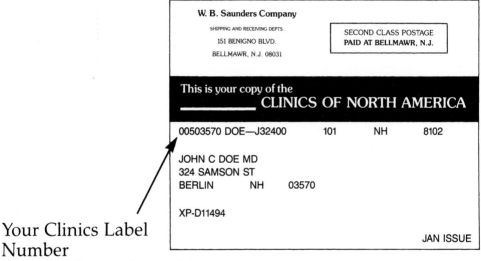

W. B. Saunders Company

SHIPPING AND RECEIVING DEPTS.
151 BENIGNO BLVD.
BELLMAWR, N.J. 08031

SECOND CLASS POSTAGE
PAID AT BELLMAWR, N.J.

This is your copy of the
——————— CLINICS OF NORTH AMERICA

00503570 DOE—J32400   101   NH   8102

JOHN C DOE MD
324 SAMSON ST
BERLIN   NH   03570

XP-D11494

JAN ISSUE

Your Clinics Label Number
Copy it exactly or send your label along with your address to:
W.B. Saunders Company, Customer Service
Orlando, FL 32887-4800
Call Toll Free 1-800-654-2452

Please allow four to six weeks for delivery of new subscriptions and for processing address changes.